TRY THESE IF

YOU WANT

TO HAVE

AMAZING

SEX

POSITIONS

THAT WILL

BLOW YOUR MIND

AND TAKE YOU

TO DIZZYING NEW

HEIGHTS OF SEXUAL

PLEASURE

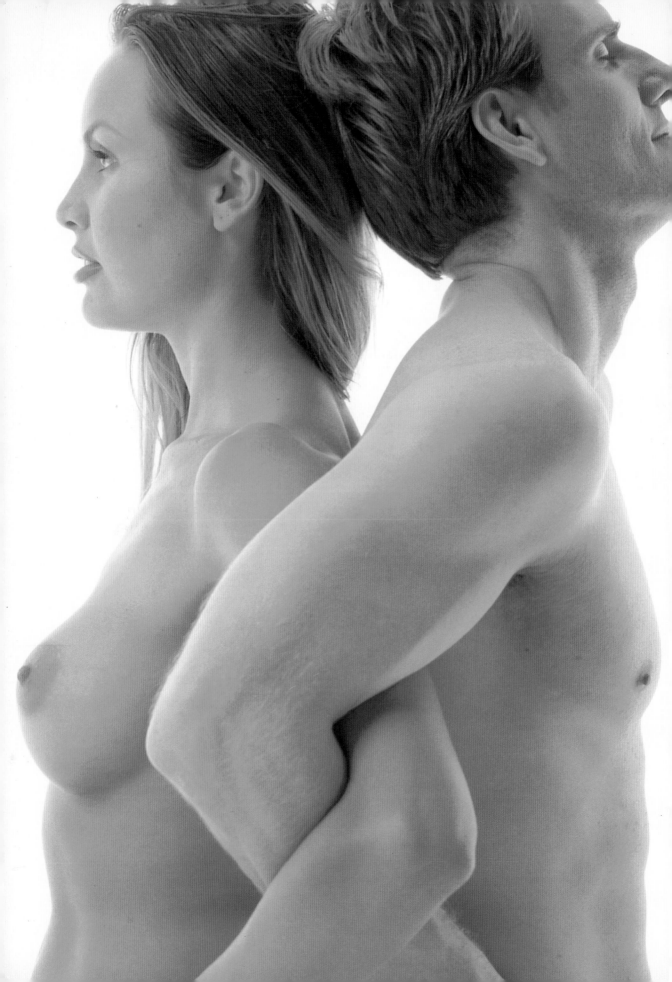

CARLTON
BOOKS

TRY THESE IF
YOU WANT
TO HAVE
AMAZING
SEX
POSITIONS
THAT WILL
BLOW YOUR MIND
AND TAKE YOU
TO DIZZYING NEW
HEIGHTS OF SEXUAL
PLEASURE

RICHARD EMERSON

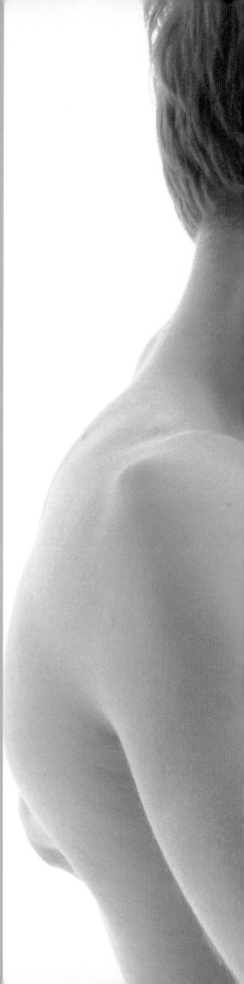

THIS IS A CARLTON BOOK

This edition published in 2018 by Carlton Books Limited.
First published as *The Best Sex You'll Ever Have!* in 2001 by
Carlton Books Limited, a division of the Carlton Publishing Group.
20 Mortimer Street, London W1T 3JW

A CIP catalogue record for this book is available from the
British Library

ISBN 978 1 78739 043 0

Printed in Hong Kong

Neither the author nor the publisher can accept responsibility
for any accident, injury or damage that results from using the
ideas, information or advice offered in this book.

The information in this book is for information only.
The advice on contraception and all other aspects of sexual
health is not intended as a substitute for the advice and
guidance of a qualified health professional. Anyone who
is concerned about a sexual or other health issue, problem
or concern should consult a doctor. If you are pregnant or
suffering from a skin condition or other medical ailment,
consult a qualified aromatherapist about suitable massage
oils you can use.

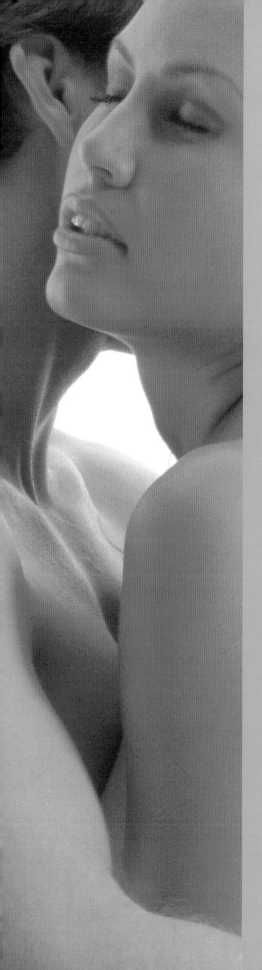

CONTENTS

INTRODUCTION

THE HUMAN BODY is a magical sexual adventure playground, full of secret wonders and delights that can lift you and your partner to towering heights of erotic fulfilment. Our skin is covered with highly sensitive nerve endings that can deliver a powerful sexual charge, when stimulated in the right way. The areas most easily aroused are the sex organs, the man's penis and testicles, and the woman's vulva and vagina, followed in sensitivity by the secondary sexual zones – breasts, nipples, thighs and buttocks.

Many people find that it can be powerfully arousing when other areas of the body are stimulated – the earlobes, the nape of the neck, the back of the knees and the toes, to name but a few. Discovering your most sensitive areas, and those of your partner, and learning how to excite them sexually, can arouse you in ways you never thought possible.

Yet, the most powerful sexual organ of all is the human mind. And it needs to be stimulated, too, with lots of variety and plenty of new ideas to pep up your partner and spice up your love life. That's where this book can help. On the following pages you'll find tips and techniques that you can try out to add more zest to your sexual quests, and lots of sex positions – some drawn from the teachings of ancient oriental masters of the erotic.

In the West, the standard pose for sexual intercourse, with the man lying on top of his partner with his body between her legs, is called the 'missionary position'. Some people think it is the only 'normal' position to adopt. In fact there are hundreds of positions, each one with an infinite number of subtle variations. And they're all great fun! It was the amorous Polynesian natives of the South Pacific islands who invented the term 'missionary position', after seeing European missionaries making love in this way. The inquisitive natives thought the Western way was rather quaint and amusing, but deadly dull. Their favoured pose for intercourse was with the woman squatting over her partner, where she could control the angle, depth and pace of penetration.

As the many hundreds of seafarers who visited these sun-drenched islands were to discover to their great delight, the uninhibited islanders were happy and eager to try out new ideas, when suggested. Sitting, standing, swinging from the palm trees, there was nothing the fertile imaginations of the lithe and golden-tanned Polynesians would not dream up in their search for the ultimate erotic experience. No wonder the browbeaten crew of HMS Bounty decided to mutiny after they were forced to leave this tropical sexual paradise.

No one is standing over you with a whip (unless you want them to), so enjoy yourself. Trial and error and plenty of practice are the best ways to find out what works for you. You don't have to attempt all the positions. But you should find something here to bring a sparkle to your eyes, colour to your cheeks and generally tickle your fancy. As a sage once remarked: 'When sex is good it's very good, but when it's bad – it's still pretty good.'

BE A SEXUAL EXPLORER

You're about to begin one of the most pleasurable voyages of discovery you will ever experience. Enjoy the ride – and hold on tight as the waves start to rock you.

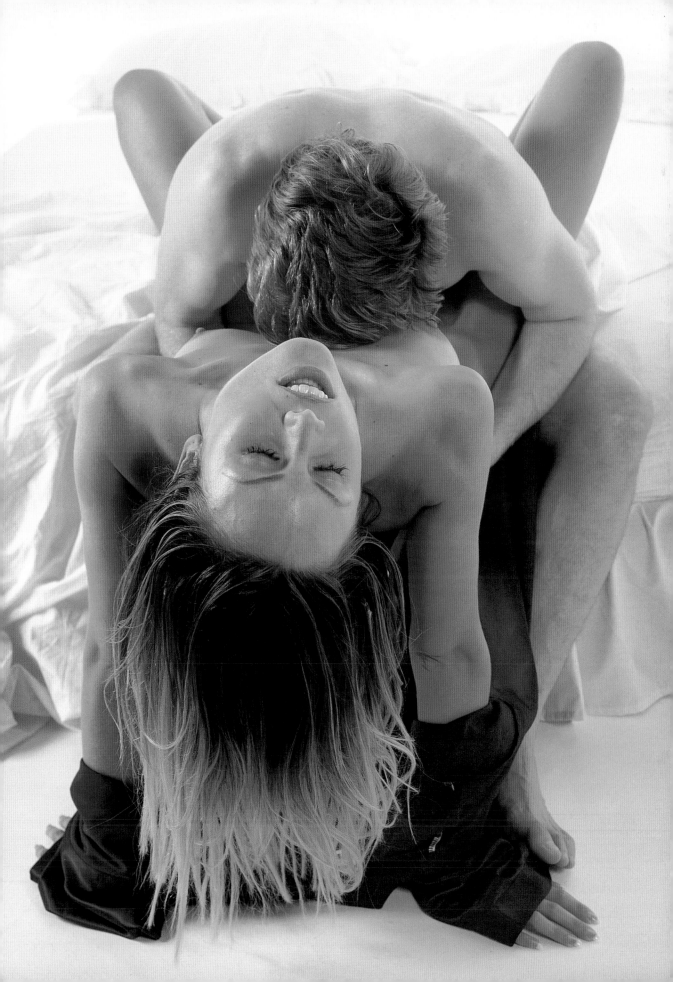

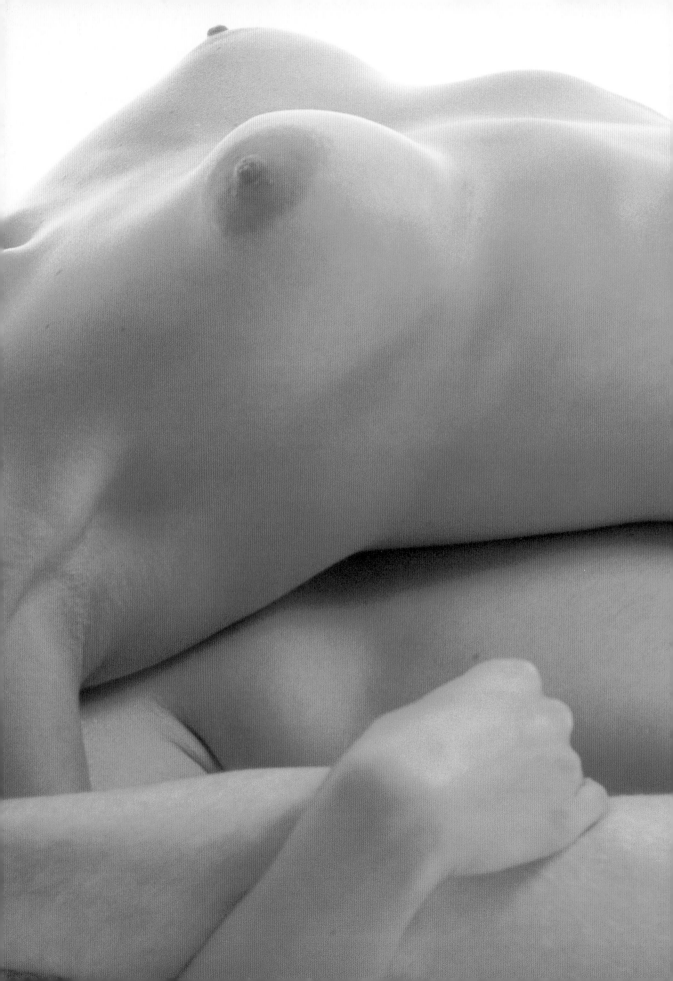

'A man on a date wonders if he'll get lucky.

A woman already knows ...'

MONICA PIPER

THE
SEXUAL
WOMAN

A WOMAN'S SEX DRIVE, OR LIBIDO, IS DETERMINED BY A COMBINATION OF PHYSICAL,

EMOTIONAL AND PSYCHOLOGICAL FACTORS. TO ENJOY LOVEMAKING TO THE

FULL, SHE NEEDS TO UNCOVER HER TRUE SEXUAL NATURE.

THIS IS OFTEN A VOYAGE OF SELF-DISCOVERY – MADE EASIER WITH THE HELP

OF A THOUGHTFUL, CARING PARTNER.

SEXUAL RHYTHM

To be sexually aroused, a woman not only needs to be strongly attracted to the man she is with, she also needs to feel good about herself, to be in the right frame of mind and in an environment that is conducive to lovemaking. Once she's in the mood for sex, the time it takes for her to become aroused depends on her own unique sexual rhythm. This differs from woman to woman, and also varies according to her age, and even the time of day, week or month. For example, a woman may find that she is much more sexually responsive shortly before, or just after, menstruation.

Love and sex

Love is a powerful sexual stimulant for a woman, so her sex drive is often strongest when she first meets her lover and it is usually maintained through having regular sex. It can decrease when she has been without a partner for a while or is experiencing relationship difficulties, is ill or has undergone surgery, is stressed, tired, feeling a lack of confidence in herself for whatever reason, or through overwork, or the demands of parenting. Cultural and social factors may also play a part in this. A woman may feel sexually inhibited because of her upbringing, perhaps through being told in childhood that sex is dirty, or that it is immoral for a woman to enjoy intercourse. Concerns over pregnancy and contraception can also suppress her libido. Factors like these can make a woman lose touch with her basic sexual nature.

JUST SAY IT

Tell your partner what you like, and encourage him to spend plenty of time caressing all your erogenous zones.

fact

Using the latest medical imaging techniques (Magnetic Resonance Imaging – MRI), scientists have discovered that the vaginal wall lengthens by as much as 75 per cent during intercourse.

EROGENOUS ZONES

The most sexually sensitive areas of a woman's body are called the erogenous zones. When stimulated, for example by being kissed or caressed by a lover, they can cause her to become sexually aroused. Apart from the genitals, her most powerful erogenous zones are her breasts, especially the nipples and the darkly pigmented areas (areolae) surrounding them. Other areas of high arousal include the inner thigh, lower back, buttocks, lower abdomen, especially the fleshy pubic mound (mons pubis) directly in front of the genitals, and the perineum, the area of skin between the genitals and the anus. Potentially, however, all parts of the female body are erogenous zones; for instance, a woman may go wild if a man kisses her neck or ears.

The vagina

The external genitals are known, collectively, as the vulva and lie between the pubic mound and the perineum. The parts of a woman's genitals that are most important for sexual arousal are the vagina, an elastic, muscular tube that opens to the outside and holds the man's erect penis during intercourse, and a very sensitive structure called the clitoris. One part of the vagina, the G-spot, is particularly sensitive. It is located on the front wall of the vagina, about 5 cm (2 in) up. When stimulated, it swells and can be felt as a bean-sized lump.

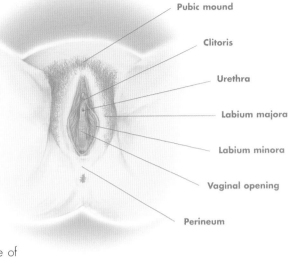

Pubic mound

Clitoris

Urethra

Labium majora

Labium minora

Vaginal opening

Perineum

The clitoris

Located at the front of the vulva, the clitoris is partly covered by a fold of skin (clitoral hood). Although only the tip (glans) of the clitoris is visible, this is just a small part of a much larger structure. It is made of erectile tissue that swells with blood when a woman is aroused, and is well supplied with nerve endings. For some women, it is too sensitive for direct stimulation and indirect friction needs to be applied to the clitoral hood or the surrounding area.

The labia

The clitoral hood is connected to two fleshy folds of skin, the outer lips (labia majora), enclosing a more delicate pair of inner lips (labia minora). These inner lips surround a moist region, the vestibule, which includes the urinary and vaginal openings. The labia minora vary in size between individuals and with age and are either covered by, or protrude beyond, the outer labia. These are all perfectly normal variations. They re-join at the back of the vulva to form the fourchette.

EXPLORE YOUR BODY

To discover your sexual nature, use a mirror to study your body as you try out different ways to stimulate yourself. You'll develop a clearer idea of your sexual anatomy and find the most effective ways to get aroused.

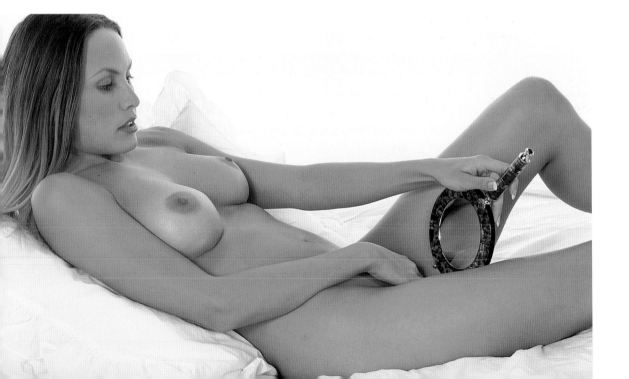

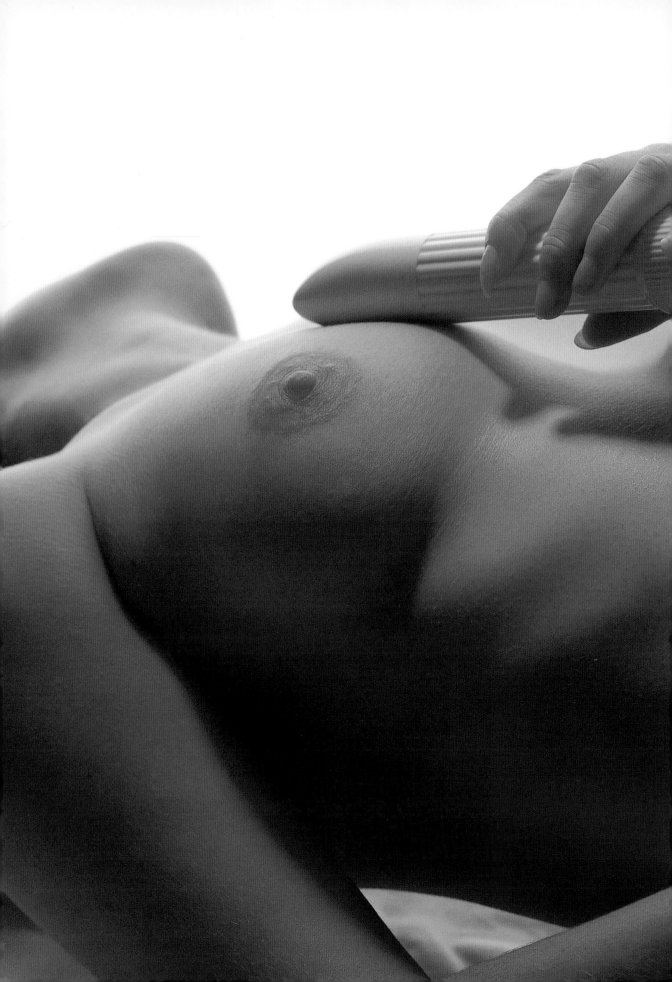

EXCITEMENT PHASE

The physical changes that signal arousal in a woman are not so apparent as in a man, whose erect penis is a good indicator of his sexual feelings. Nevertheless, a woman must be sexually aroused for her vagina to be open and moist enough to allow comfortable penetration. During sex, a woman's body goes through four distinct phases. First, during the excitement phase, her pulse and breathing rate increase, breasts enlarge slightly, nipples grow erect, the areolae darken, vagina and clitoris become engorged with blood and the clitoris becomes erect. The vagina releases a lubricating fluid to make intercourse more comfortable, which is felt as moistness around the vaginal opening, and her chest may show a characteristic 'sex flush'.

PLATEAU PHASE

Sexual excitement heightens until the woman reaches the plateau phase, during which her state of arousal remains at the same level for a time. Throughout this phase, the lower part of her vagina narrows and the upper part balloons, becoming longer and wider, the labia minora darken and the clitoris shortens and withdraws under its hood.

FEMALE ORGASM

The woman's arousal then climbs again until it peaks with a sexual climax or orgasm. On average, a woman needs around 13 minutes of arousal before having an orgasm (ten minutes longer than a man) and some women may need longer. Her orgasm can last up to a minute, but most orgasms usually go on for five to ten seconds. As she climaxes, rhythmic contractions begin in the lower part of her vagina and spread through her reproductive organs. Her body becomes rigid, her lower abdominal muscles contract, her back arches and her toes curl. The sex flush spreads over her skin, accompanied by intense feelings of pleasure and wellbeing. She may moan or scream, laugh or cry, or simply remain quiet. Responses are infinite. Some women release a special fluid during orgasm, but its function is unknown.

MULTIPLE ORGASMS

Orgasm is followed by a winding-down stage, known as the refractory phase, when the woman's body reverts to its pre-arousal state and she feels a deep sense of relaxation and contentment. In many women, if stimulation continues shortly after orgasm they will return to the plateau phase, without entering resolution, and may swiftly climax again. This

tip

Some women do not produce enough natural lubrication, which can lead to painful sex, especially in later life, and they may need to use artificial forms. Special lubricating gels are available from pharmacies.

fact

The clitoris will return to its pre-excitement state within 20 seconds of orgasm and can often be re-stimulated to bring a woman to orgasm again.

ENJOY YOURSELF

OPPOSITE: *You're the best person to know what turns you on, so try different forms of stimulation; a vibrator produces mind-blowing sensations when applied to various parts of the body.*

can be repeated many times (more than ten times is not unknown) when it is called multiple orgasm. But some women find their genitals are much too sensitive to be stimulated again at this stage and up to 30 minutes must elapse before they can be re-aroused. Nevertheless, the refractory phase is much shorter in females than in males, so most women may be capable of several orgasms during sex.

fact

Women who masturbated as teenagers are often more in tune with their sexual responses and find it easier to climax during sex with a partner.

STIMULATION METHODS

Women usually achieve orgasm through stimulation of the clitoral area, or the vaginal opening, or the vaginal wall itself, either by the action of their partner's penis during penetrative sex, or by manual stimulation, or their partner's lips and tongue during oral sex. By trial and error, a woman can discover whether she gets most satisfaction from, for example, penile stimulation of the vagina, or manual stimulation of the clitoris, or a combination of these. Many women say that a clitoral orgasm is more intense and a vaginal orgasm more emotionally fulfilling – but that both are equally satisfying.

bedroom assertiveness

It's important to discover your sexual likes and dislikes and to communicate them to your partner. This is called being sexually assertive and ensures that your sexual needs are regarded as equal to his. However, for the sake of harmony in a relationship, try to make your feelings known without making your partner feel that you're putting him down. For example:

- **Do be receptive to new ideas from your partner and suggest your own, too.**

- **Do say if you're in the mood for sex. A woman's libido is as powerful as a man's and there's nothing unfeminine about taking the initiative. Don't feel pressurized into sex if you're not feeling sexy and be tolerant if he is not in the mood.**

- **Do discuss menstruation with your partner. You may feel self-conscious about making love at this time and many men are uncomfortable with the idea and may prefer to abstain for religious, cultural or personal, reasons.**

- **Do speak up if you don't like something your partner is doing, but try to be tactful. Rather than the negative 'Don't do that!,' try a more positive approach, such as 'I'd much rather you did this ...'**

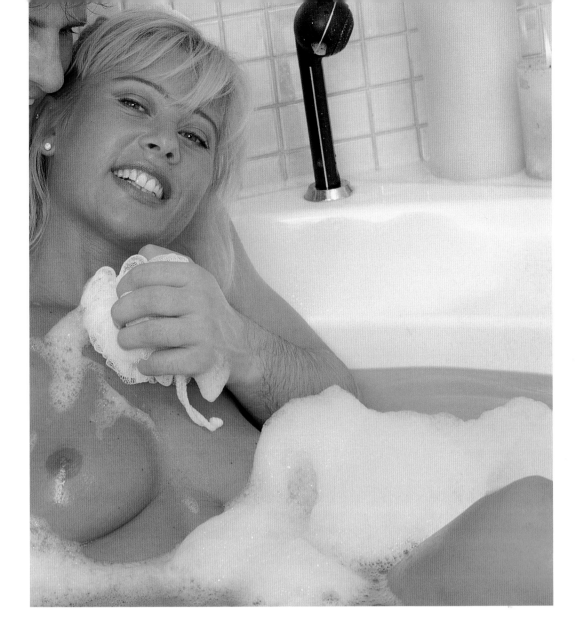

AGE ADVANTAGES

In general, women take longer than men to climax but are capable of more orgasms. This may lead to problems of sexual incompatibility but these can be avoided, provided the man ensures that his partner is in the mood for love, and fully aroused and close to climaxing before concentrating on his own sexual satisfaction. Woman often find their sex drive increases as they get older and they become capable of having more orgasms more often. Some say they feel sexiest, and have the shortest arousal time, from their late thirties to forties. This may be because a woman needs time to discover her sexual responses. Also, by her thirties she is more likely to be in a stable relationship with a man who has taken time to learn her sexual needs. The difference between male and female arousal times narrows with age.

BATH-TIME FUN

Sharing a bath is a great way to encourage your partner to touch and explore your body in a relaxed, unpressured environment.

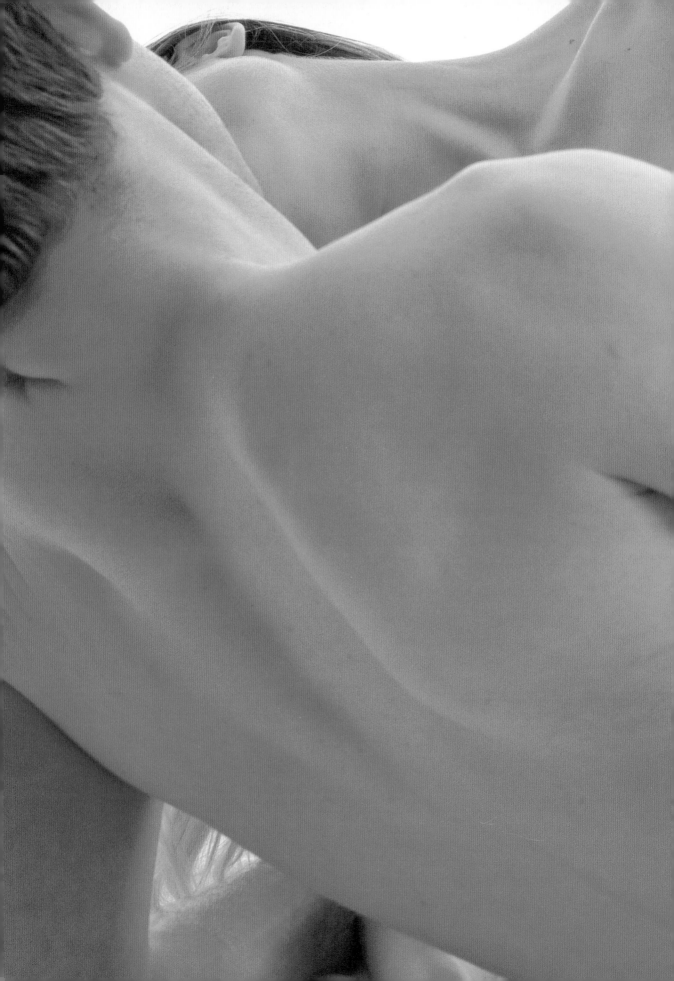

THE SEXUAL MAN

2

MANY PARTS OF A MAN'S BODY RESPOND TO SEXUAL STIMULATION, AND NOT

JUST THE GENITAL AREA, BUT HE MAY NEED TO BE ENCOURAGED TO LOOK FOR THEM.

BY LEARNING TO DERIVE PLEASURE FROM NON-GENITAL AREAS OF HIS BODY,

A MAN CAN PROLONG HIS LOVEMAKING AND GAIN MORE ENJOYMENT

FROM HIS SEXUAL EXPERIENCES.

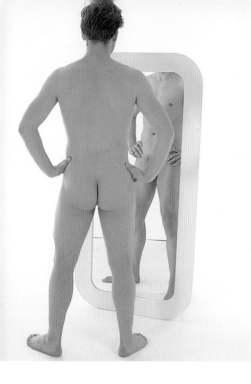

fact

**As a man approaches orgasm,
he reaches a point of no return
called 'ejaculatory inevitability'
when he cannot stop himself.
A woman, however, can be
distracted from her orgasm
right up to the last moment.**

MALE SEX DRIVE

For a man, sexual arousal is mainly triggered by sensory signals: the look, feel, scent and voice of a woman being the most important ones. Erotic images in a film or magazine can swiftly spark a man's desires, even if he hadn't been thinking about sex beforehand. In contrast to his partner, emotional rapport and romantic atmosphere play lesser roles in stirring his passion. Nevertheless, psychological factors do play an important part in the male libido. Fatigue, stress, depression and anxiety can all affect a man's sex drive negatively, even leading to an inability to achieve or maintain an erection (erectile dysfunction or impotence).

SEXUAL VARIETY

Whereas love is a strong sexual stimulant for women, novelty and variety are more important factors for men. To remain strongly sexually attracted to his partner, a man may need to have a regular change of stimulation, for example, by trying a range of sexual practices, positions or locations, using fantasy role play or sex toys, or by seeing his partner in different kinds of sexy clothes.

EROGENOUS ZONES

Unlike a woman, whose entire body is a potential erogenous zone, a man's sexual feelings are mostly centred on his genitals. As a consequence, sexual stimulation can all-too-quickly lead to orgasm before he has satisfied his partner. However, if a man is encouraged to discover his non-genital erogenous zones it can help him to delay reaching his sexual climax too quickly, while still deriving much enjoyment from lovemaking. For example, his neck, earlobes, navel, back, chest, nipples, buttocks and feet are all well served with nerve endings that respond to the feminine touch.

Anal arousal

Some of the most sensitive areas of a man's body are those closest to the genitals, such as the lower abdomen and inner thighs. An often-neglected erogenous zone is the perineum, the area of skin between the scrotum and the anus. The anus itself is probably the most sexually sensitive area of a man's body, other than his genitals. A woman's light touch on his buttock cheeks and circling the rim of the anus is a powerful turn-on for many men.

MALE GENITALS

A man's genitals are mostly external. The most
important structures for sexual arousal are the
penis, a long tube containing cylinders of erectile
tissue; and the testicles, two oval, ball-shaped
structures covered by a sac of skin called the
scrotum. In uncircumcized men, a collar of
skin, known as the foreskin, partly covers the
tip of the penis. The foreskin rolls back to
reveal the cap-shaped glans. (In circumcized
men, the foreskin is removed.) On the underside
of the penis, where the glans meets the shaft, is a
small flap of skin called the frenulum. During arousal
the penis hardens and lengthens. In general, the larger
the penis when flaccid, the smaller the increase in size when
erect. In contrast, a small penis can increase many times in length.

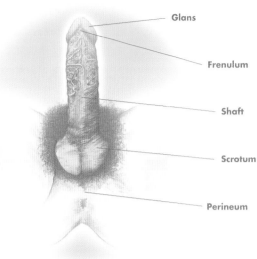

Glans

Frenulum

Shaft

Scrotum

Perineum

All parts of the genitals are sensitive, but the degree of sensitivity varies
from man to man. Some men prefer their partner to pay particular
attention to the shaft of the penis, whereas others enjoy having their
scrotum fondled. When stroking a man's penis, women are often too
gentle, worried that they might hurt him. In fact, men often prefer more
friction than women realize. The best way to find out where, and how,
a man wants to be stimulated is by experiment. You may also like to
watch him as he pleasures himself (page 55)

TEASE YOURSELF

*You can gain more from sex
by discovering non-genital areas
of arousal and encouraging
your partner to stimulate them
during lovemaking.*

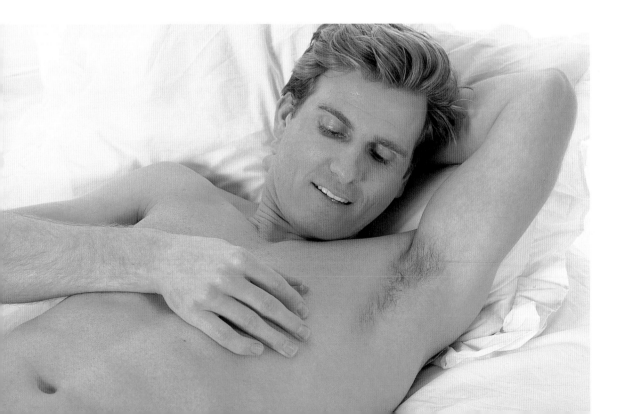

coming together

A man may feel a sexual failure unless he and his partner climax together. Few couples achieve this every time, and many rarely manage it. As long as both partners are satisfied, it doesn't really matter at what stage they climax. If simultaneous orgasms are important to you, however, the following tips may help:

- **A man can use his hands, mouth and imagination to bring his partner close to orgasm before penetration.**

- **He can ensure his partner has already had at least one orgasm. Re-arousal is quicker in a woman, so her subsequent orgasm may coincide with his.**

- **He or she can apply pressure to the top of the penis, just below the glans, or to its base to reduce the erection temporarily and so delay ejaculation (see page 114).**

EXCITEMENT PHASE

A man, too, goes through four distinct phases of arousal. First, the excitement phase, when his heart and breathing rate rise dramatically, especially when performing strong pelvic thrusting movements. His penis reaches full extension and gets almost painfully hard, his glans darkens in colour, while his scrotal skin tightens. A few drops of semen (pre-ejaculate) may seep from the urethral opening at the tip of the penis at any stage before orgasm. For this reason, if you are using any form of barrier contraception, such as a condom, it must be in place before the penis is inserted into the vagina.

PLATEAU PHASE

As sexual stimulation increases, a man soon reaches his plateau phase, and may swiftly build to a climax unless he can delay or extend this phase. This usually involves a combination of techniques (see 'Coming Together', left). One way for the man to slow or stop penile stimulation is by withdrawing his penis from his partner's vagina and stimulating her by hand until she is close to having an orgasm. Another way is to contract his pubococcygeal (PB) muscles – the ones he uses to stop himself urinating. He may also think 'unsexy' thoughts, or use the 'Squeeze' technique, page 114, to dampen his ardour.

MALE ORGASM

As the man approaches orgasm, his muscles begin to go rigid with tension and his face contorts into a grimace. The intense feeling of pleasure experienced at orgasm is usually accompanied by ejaculation. Muscles in the urethra (the tube that carries urine out of the body) and around the base of the penis contract rhythmically to eject semen in a series of powerful spurts that steadily grow weaker. The muscles of his lower abdomen contract in waves and his thigh muscles tense up. Like his partner, a pink flush may spread over his body and he may call out, although some men are incapable of making a sound. Male orgasm usually lasts four to ten seconds, and rarely longer than 15 seconds.

REFRACTORY PHASE

Orgasm is followed by the refractory phase, when the man's body reverts to its pre-arousal state. In contrast to the plateau phase, the refractory phase is much longer in men than in women. Even a young man may have to wait 20 minutes or more before he is capable of another erection, while an older man may need to wait several hours.

A man may feel an intense drowsiness after orgasm, which he finds hard to resist. While men are naturally made this way, this is a potential cause of conflict between the sexes as women often want their lovemaking to end with a cuddle and a few loving words – signs they are loved as well as desired. For the sake of the relationship, a man should try to resist his fatigue, or at least take his partner in his arms, before sleep eventually overcomes him.

AGE AND SEX

A man's sex drive is strongest in his teens, when his desire for sex is greatest and the time it takes him to become re-aroused after orgasm is shortest. This is usually a time when he'll have few opportunities for sex with a female, so he'll probably experience his first orgasms through adolescent masturbation. As a young man gets a 'sexual high' so quickly and easily by masturbating – often several times in a day – he has little incentive to learn how to postpone it. So, when he eventually forms a sexual relationship with a woman, he may have difficulty in adapting to his partner's slower sexual response times.

From his early twenties onward, a man notices a slow, but steady, increase in the time it takes for him to get aroused and re-aroused. This is no bad thing. Along with a reduced sense of urgency comes a greater willingness to make sex last longer and be emotionally more rewarding. A man's growing patience should encourage him to take care to ensure his partner is sexually satisfied, too.

safety first

Although an erect penis seems hard and resilient, its blood vessels and other structures are vulnerable to fracture. Take care not to make any sudden or extreme changes of position, especially when the penis is deep inside the vagina, that may cause the penis to bend abnormally.

fact

A man may climax without ejaculating – especially if he has already ejaculated once during a session of lovemaking.

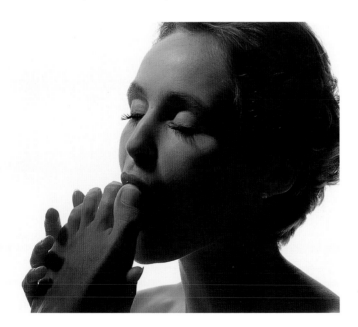

TOE TURN-ON

The feet are extremely sensitive, but an often-neglected area of the body. Sucking the big toe, in particular, can be a powerful turn-on for many men.

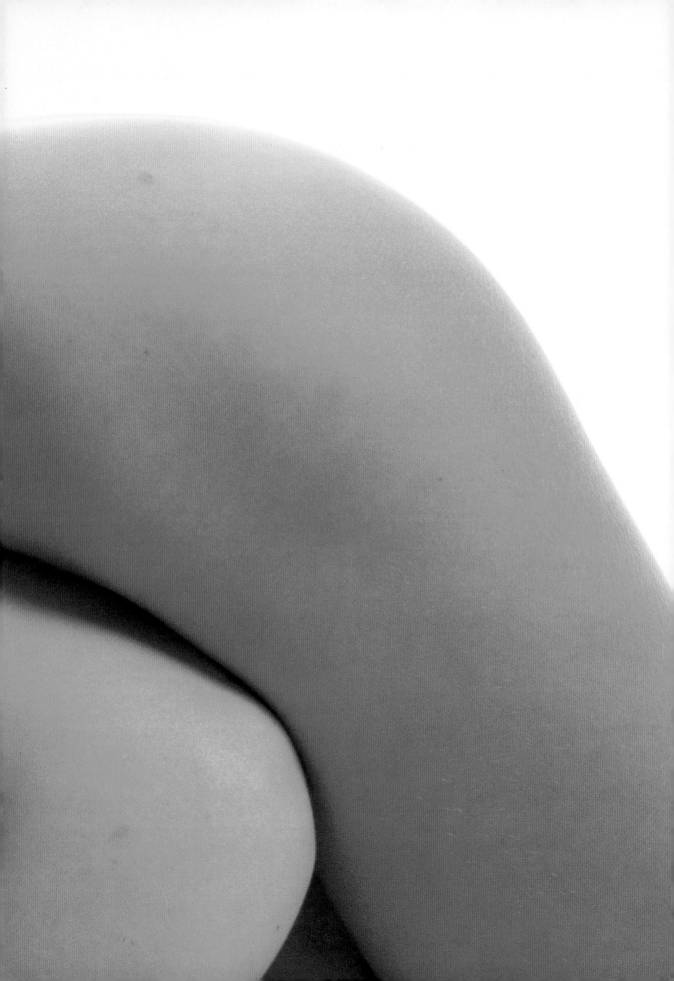

3

FIT FOR LOVE

REGULAR EXERCISE CAN GIVE COUPLES THE STAMINA AND SUPPLENESS THEY NEED

TO EXPLORE THE ADVENTUROUS SIDE OF THEIR SEXUAL NATURE. IT IMPROVES MUSCLE

TONE, POSTURE AND SHAPE, WHICH CONTRIBUTES TO A BETTER SELF-IMAGE,

AND PROMOTES A GREATER RANGE OF PELVIC MOVEMENTS – IDEAL FOR

ENTHUSIASTIC LOVEMAKING.

SEXUAL FITNESS

Sex is a highly physical activity so, to get the most out of it, couples should aim to enhance their sexual fitness through regular exercise. This will ensure that those muscles and joints that work hardest during sex have the strength, suppleness and mobility to cope with any position the couple wish to try without the risk of premature fatigue, aches, pain or – heaven forbid – injury. It is particularly important when practising the more active or athletic positions shown in this book.

Nothing deflates a moment of passion faster than an attack of cramp, and this might even deter a couple from ever being sexually adventurous again. A well-planned fitness regime should include regular stamina-building exercises like brisk walking, cycling, jogging or swimming. Just three 30-minute sessions of such activities each week can make a big difference to sexual stamina and help ensure that men and women get the maximum enjoyment from their lovemaking.

SEXERCISE

The exercises in this chapter are for both sexes and are designed to condition the muscles of the buttocks, thighs, abdomen and lower back that are used actively during sex but may be neglected in other fitness regimes. They improve strength, tone and joint mobility, help you to bear your partner's weight, and make it easier to do the more tiring positions – especially those involving squatting and thrusting movements. What's more, they will allow you to move smoothly and with control, and to extend your range of movement. Ideally, you should do some or all of these exercises at least three days a week, spaced at intervals.

Love muscles

An area of the body that benefits most from strengthening exercises is the pelvic floor. This is the collection of muscles, ligaments and other structures that support the bladder, urethra, rectum and reproductive organs. To find them, simply pretend you have a full bladder but are trying to prevent yourself from urinating. The contraction you feel indicates your pelvic floor. A strong pelvic floor enables a man to delay ejaculation and a woman to tighten her pelvic muscles around her partner's penis to increase the stimulation they both receive during sex. Each day, contract your pelvic floor ten times quickly, then ten times slowly. You can do this anywhere (even in public) as no one will notice.

Studies show that people who exercise moderately, at least three times a week, are more sexually active and have a better self-image than those who do little exercise. More sex is not necessarily the same as better sex, but women who tone their abdominal muscles and strengthen their pelvic floor find their orgasms are stronger and more intense, and they climax more quickly.

The warm-up

Choose a warm, draught-free room to exercise in and remember to wear loose, comfortable clothes. Before you start these 'sexercises', always warm up thoroughly first by having a hot bath or shower, or spend five minutes walking on the spot, swinging your arms around, or step up and down on a step or stair. This ensures your muscles and joints are warm and mobile, so reducing the risk of injury. While exercising, breathe smoothly and evenly, and never hold your breath. Keep your back straight and stretched and your chin tucked in. These exercises are suitable for men and woman and should be carried out in addition to (not instead of) an all-round fitness programme.

safety first

- **Don't attempt these exercises if you're overweight, pregnant, or suffering back pain or any other medical condition. A doctor or other relevant health professional can recommend a suitable exercise programme for you.**

- **Stop at once if any action causes pain.**

- **Don't force a movement to the point of pain.**

- **You can exercise in bare feet, but trainers (sneakers) with a good grip and an exercise mat are recommended.**

- **Do keep your actions smooth; avoid sudden, jerky or rapid movements as these can lead to injury.**

- **Do exercise in a warm, draught-free room and wear clothes that will not restrict your movements.**

- **Stop at once if you experience breathlessness, heart palpitations, nausea or pain in the chest, arms or jaw.**

- **Don't exercise if you have a cough, cold or other sign of active infection.**

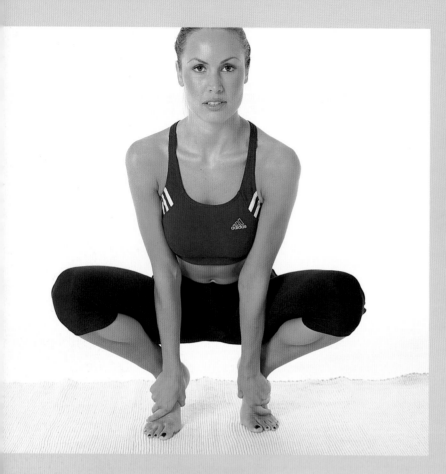

PELVIC SQUATS

Squat down, keeping your feet wide enough apart to support you safely and facing forward. With your arms pointing down, holding onto your feet if you need extra support, relax your pelvic floor. Take five short in-breaths, tightening your pelvic floor steadily with each breath. Now give five short out-breaths, steadily relaxing your pelvic floor. Repeat ten times.

STRETCHING THE INNER THIGHS

Place a cushion (pillow) on the floor and sit on the edge, facing away from it. Place the soles of your feet together, breathe in and grasping your ankles, pull your feet up as close to your body as is comfortable. Breathe out, and ease your knees as far down to the floor as they will comfortably go, then release. Repeat ten times.

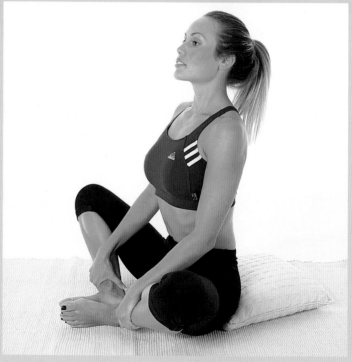

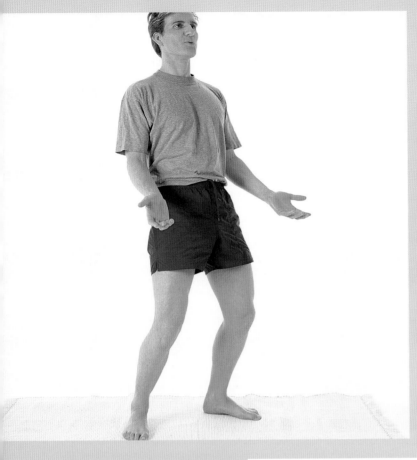

PELVIC SWING

Stand with your feet shoulder-width apart, facing forward, your knees slightly flexed and your arms loosely by your sides. Breathe in as you draw your pelvis back; breathe out as you swing your pelvis forward, bringing your arms up at the same time. Repeat ten times.

PELVIC CIRCLES

Stand with your feet shoulder-width apart, facing forward, and knees slightly flexed. Place your hands on the sides of your hips. Breathe in and out smoothly as you describe wide circles with your hips, ten times clockwise, then ten times anticlockwise.

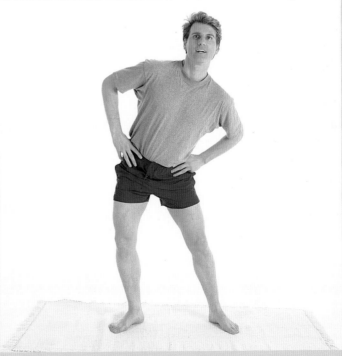

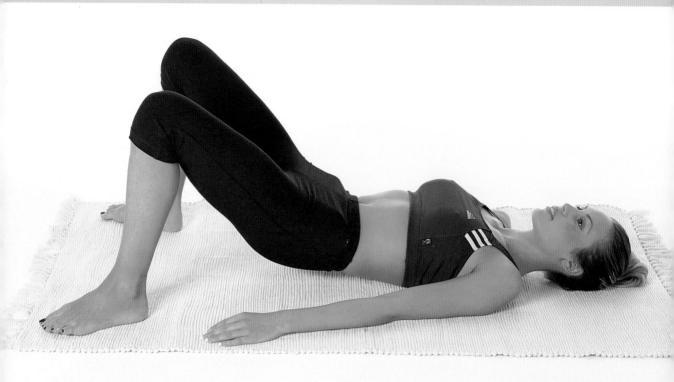

TUMMY TONER

ABOVE LEFT: *Lie with your back pressed to the floor and your arms loosely by your sides. With your knees raised, breathe in as you pull your tummy in and tilt your pelvis upward slightly.*

RIGHT: *Breathe out and stretch your hands toward your knees, raising your head and shoulders off the floor. Repeat ten times. (Remember to keep your back flat on the floor.)*

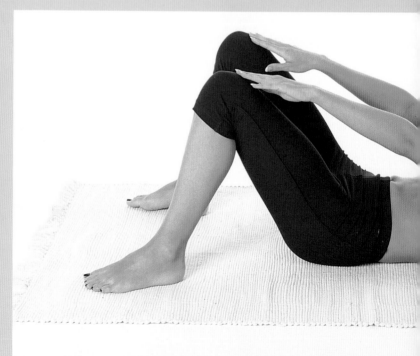

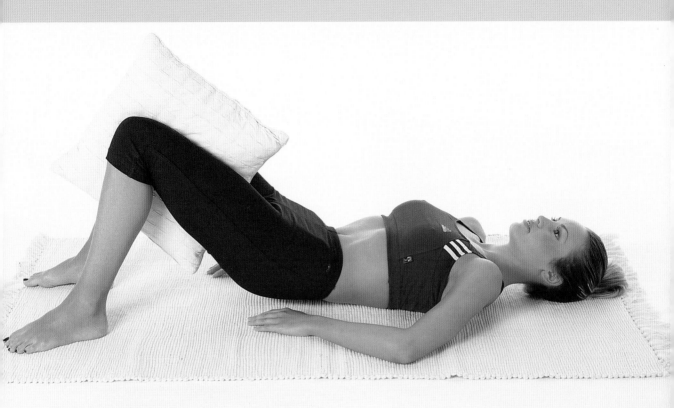

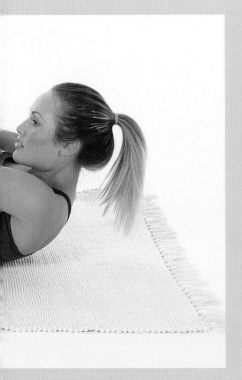

STRENGTHENING THE
INNER THIGHS

ABOVE RIGHT: *Lie on your back with your knees raised, toes pointing forward, with a cushion (pillow) pressed between your thighs and your arms loosely by your sides. Breathe in as you pull your tummy in and tilt your pelvis upward slightly. Still gripping the cushion (pillow), squeeze your knees together and then relax slightly. Breathe out. Repeat ten times.*

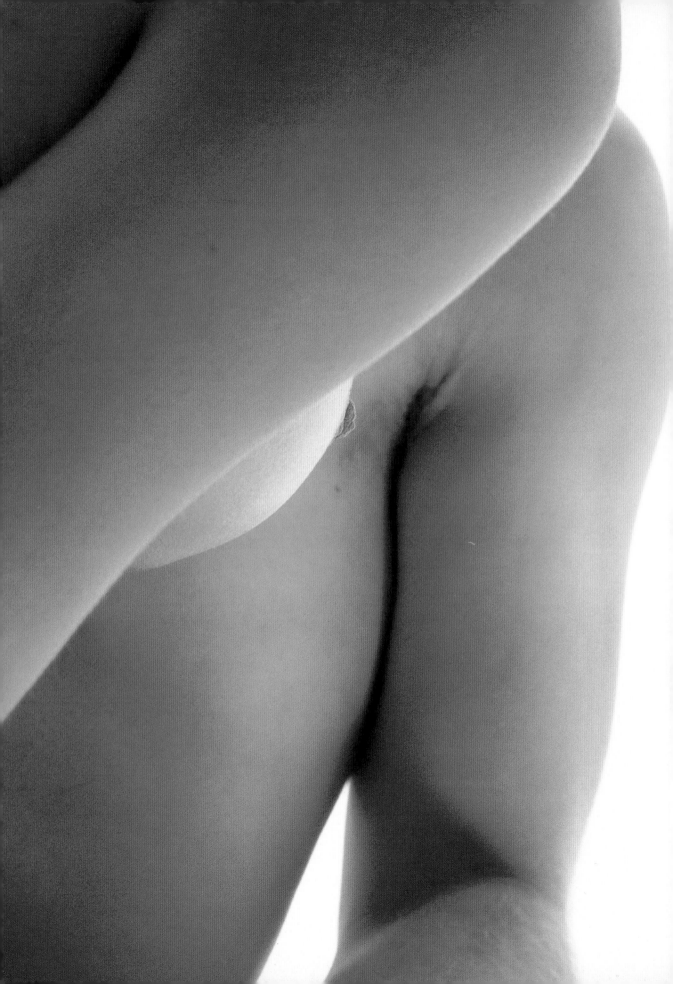

IN THE
MOOD FOR
ROMANCE

CREATING A SULTRY, SENSUAL ATMOSPHERE HELPS TO ENHANCE THE MOOD FOR LOVE

– AND LOVEMAKING. A HEADY BLEND OF ROMANCE AND SEXUAL CHEMISTRY, WITH

TWO PEOPLE ATTUNED TO EACH OTHER'S NEEDS AND DESIRES, ARE THE PERFECT

INGREDIENTS TO MAKE MAGIC.

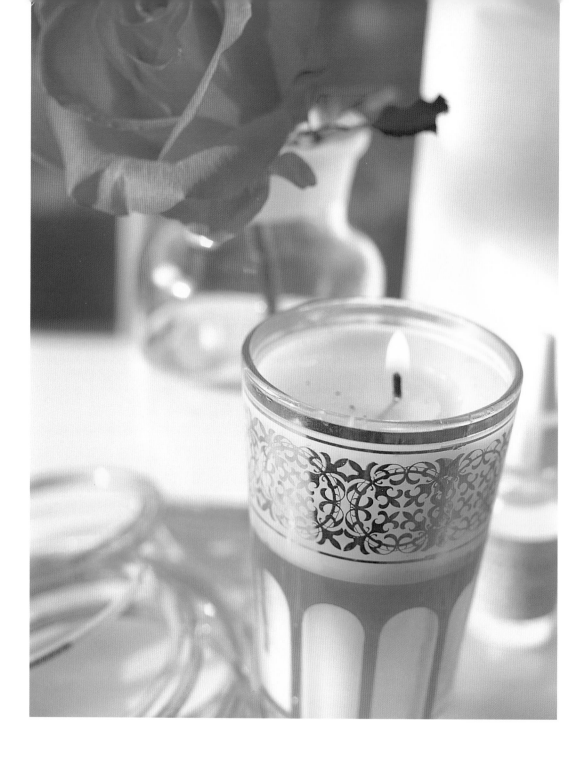

THE ART OF AROUSAL

SET THE MOOD

For a romantic evening at home, get the atmosphere right from the start. A beautiful table arrangement adds an air of intimacy and promotes togetherness.

Whether you're spending an evening with a long-established partner, or inviting a special person home for the first time, it's worth while making a little effort to create the right atmosphere for intimacy. For most women, a large helping of romance is a vital accompaniment to love. Even on a good day, when everything has gone well and she is feeling really good about herself, a woman needs a steady build-up to sex, with lots of kissing and cuddling to make her feel wanted and desired. On a day filled with frustrations, anxieties or a heavy workload, she needs even more cosseting to help her switch off and turn to thoughts of love. A man, too, needs time to unwind from his tensions and anxieties and enjoy his partner's company. By making your home a sensual oasis, cut off from the tribulations of the outside world, you can create the perfect mood for explosive lovemaking.

LOUNGE LOVING

Select a time when your lovemaking won't be disturbed. Switch on the answerphone and, if you have children, settle them in bed, or choose a time when they're staying with friends or relatives. Avoid setting a timetable; let the evening unfold as it may. A warm, unhurried bath or shower − preferably shared − is the perfect preliminary to lovemaking, washing away all the cares of the day. Soap each other all over, massaging the lather well into the muscles of your bodies and enjoy the sight and touch of each other. Continue the massage experience with oils (see pages 41 and 42) or body lotion, if liked. You can follow this up with a romantic dinner together; a glass or two of wine may help you to relax. But keep the meal light or you'll both feel too full or sleepy for sex. If you choose a simple meal and share in the preparation and cooking, you'll help to strengthen the bond between you and set the mood of sharing and giving that will enhance your lovemaking. Candlelight increases the mood, creating soft, sexy shadows that hint at intimacies to come, and scenting the room with aromatic fragrance. Ensure the room is warm enough to undress in comfort, but not so hot that you will feel sleepy. Open a window slightly to let in a little fresh air and place a bowl of water near a radiator to prevent the room getting too dry. Fresh sheets on the bed (linen or silk) and wearing exotic underwear (page 92) and scent adds to the sensual atmosphere.

LIGHT OF DESIRE

Make the most of the ambience by giving yourselves the whole evening to enjoy each other's sensuality. Curl up on a sofa to kiss and cuddle like teenagers. As you grow more aroused, slowly begin to undress each other, delighting in the look and feel of your partner's body as each new area of flesh is revealed. When the moment is right, you can transfer to the bedroom, or enjoy the change of location and continue making love in the lounge. There's a special magic to sex on a sofa, or passion on a deep-pile rug or cushions (pillows) on the floor, bathed in the cosy glow of an open fire.

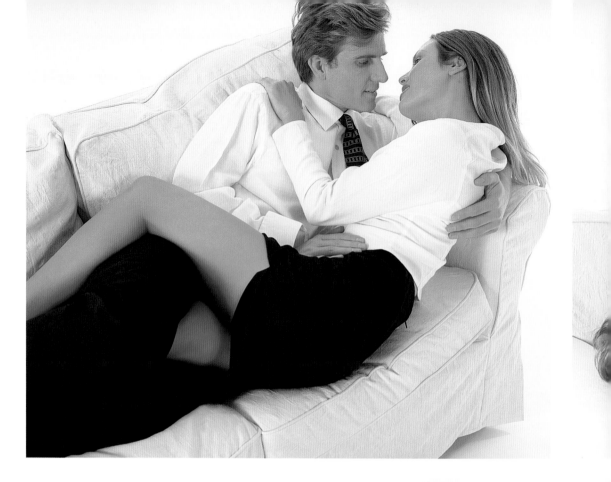

LOVING TOUCH

*Sit close together, listen to soft
music and free yourself of any sense
of urgency. Loving cuddles will soon
blossom into passion as the mood
takes over.*

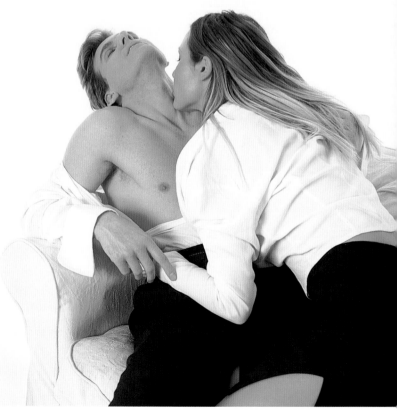

PEELING ...

*Take your time as you undress each
other. Rushing now will just make
you both fumble-fingered, so
prolong the pleasure. Undo each
fastening slowly and pay close
attention to each new area of
skin that is revealed.*

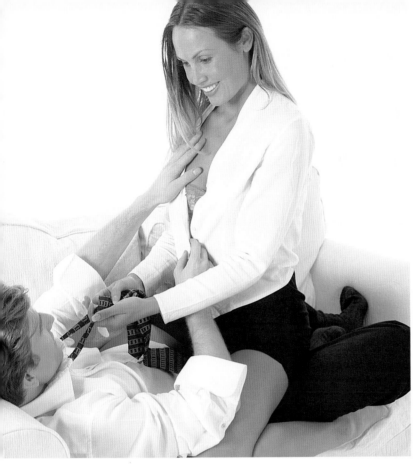

EROTIC PETTING

Don't be in too much of a hurry to strip off. Enjoy exploring each other over and under your clothes, relishing the feel of firm flesh through soft fabric.

... COMPLIMENTING

People are often self-conscious about their appearance so pay your partner compliments as you remove each item, saying how sexy he or she looks.

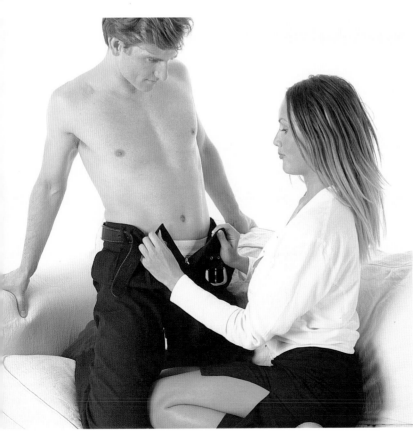

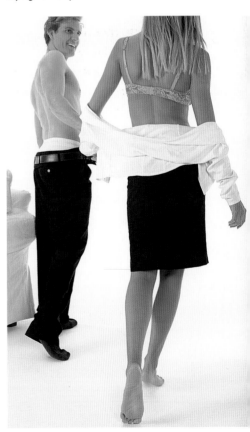

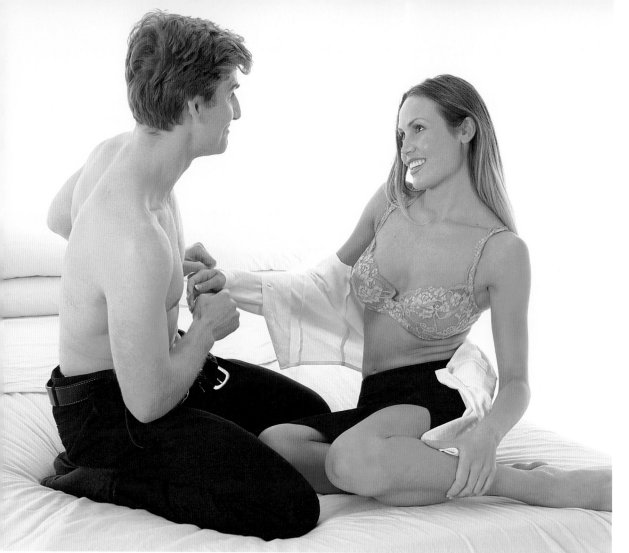

TEASING ...

Make it a game and tease your partner. Pretend to be confused about how the clothes unfasten, and 'accidentally' brush your hand against a sensitive part of their body.

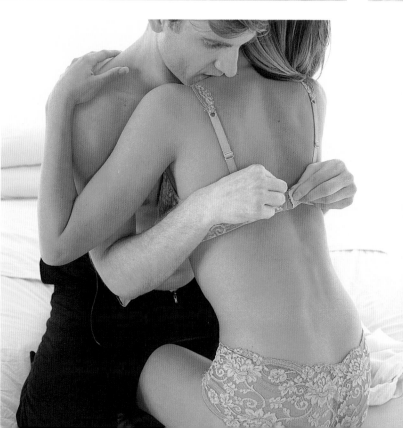

... ENCOURAGING

If your partner seems to be struggling with your bra strap, give him some encouragement – but avoid taking over. Be patient and while he's concentrating on the job in hand, lean close and whisper sexily in his ear.

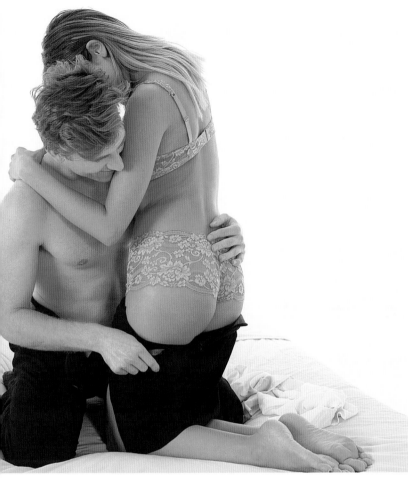

... CARESSING

Take turns to remove an item of your partner's clothing. But don't sit passively as you wait your turn. While you're being undressed, take the opportunity to kiss and caress your lover.

... EXPOSING

BOTTOM LEFT: As her breasts are exposed, pause to enjoy how they look and feel, cradling them in your hands and let your partner know how sexy she makes you feel.

... REVEALING

Knickers are the last items to remove so – no matter how aroused you are – don't rush. As you slip the soft material down over your partner's thighs you'll have plenty of other opportunities to touch, tease and tantalize.

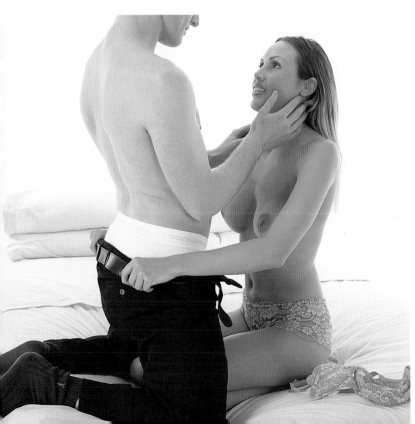

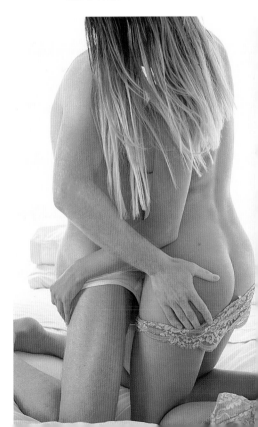

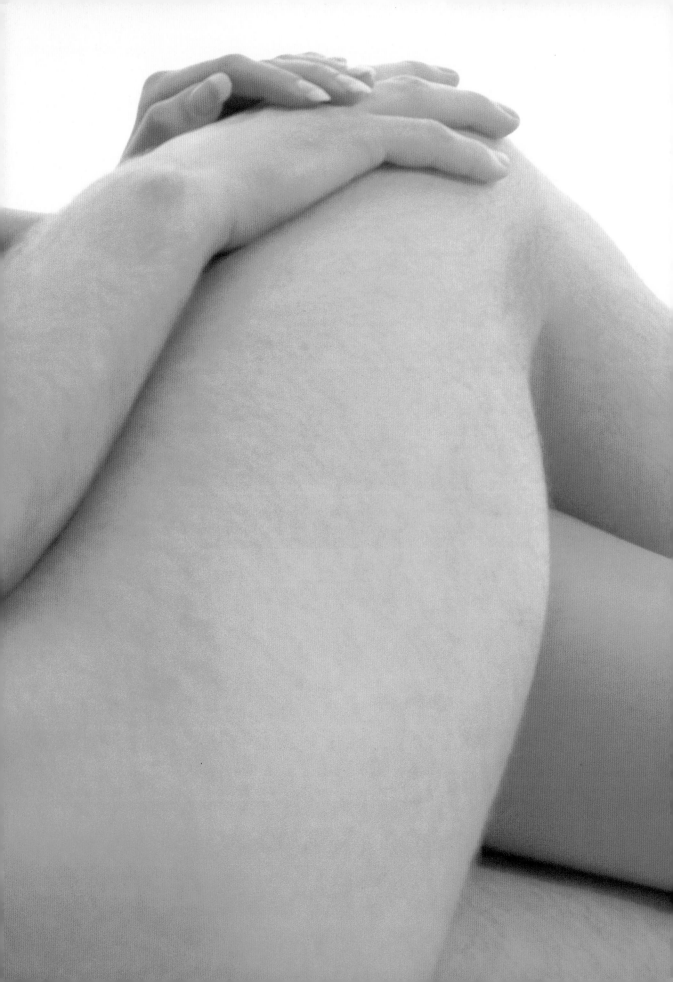

THE
TENDER
TOUCH

A SENSUAL MASSAGE PROMOTES TRUST AND COMMUNICATION IN

A RELATIONSHIP. COUPLES BECOME ATTUNED TO THEIR PARTNER'S RESPONSES AND

DISCOVER HOW TO GIVE PLEASURE IN A LOVING AND UNSELFISH WAY.

BY RECEIVING A MASSAGE THEY LEARN HOW TO LIE BACK AND SURRENDER TOTALLY

TO THEIR LOVER'S GENTLE TOUCH.

fact

Massage, petting and non-penetrative sex can relieve stress symptoms, such as anxiety and tension, and help smooth over relationship problems.

SWEEPING STROKES

Use generous, sweeping strokes, allowing your hands to fan out and maintain maximum contact with the skin. Apply firmer pressure on the forward stroke and use a light, gliding motion as you draw your hands back.

LOVING AND GIVING

A man will find that giving a woman a massage is as rewarding as receiving one. It lets him explore his partner's body and enjoy the soft feel of her skin. It's also a good way to make her feel pampered, secure and wanted in a loving and giving environment. He should be attentive to his partner's responses, using intuition to guide his hands to the areas of her body that need extra attention. For a highly arousing massage, nothing beats oiled fingertips drawn lightly over sensitive areas such as the neck or breasts. Don't limit yourself to using hands alone, but bring your lips and tongue into play, too. By giving a man an arousing massage, a woman can enjoy the feel of her partner's body, discover new areas of sensitivity and create a cosy, relaxed atmosphere for them both. She can soothe away the stresses and strains of her partner's day and get him in the mood for love.

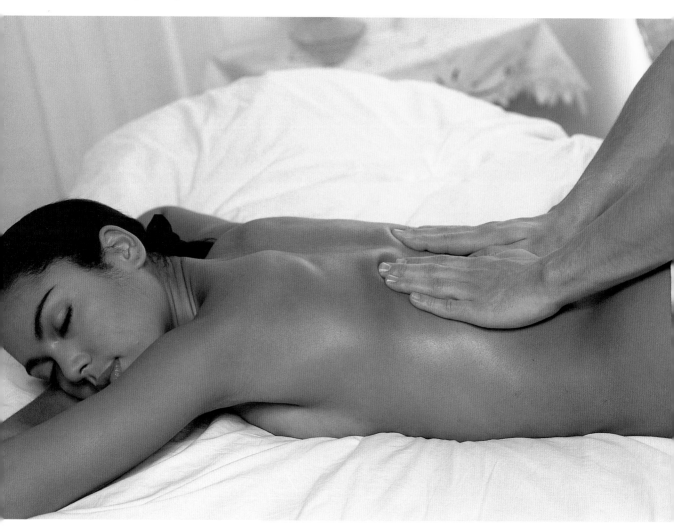

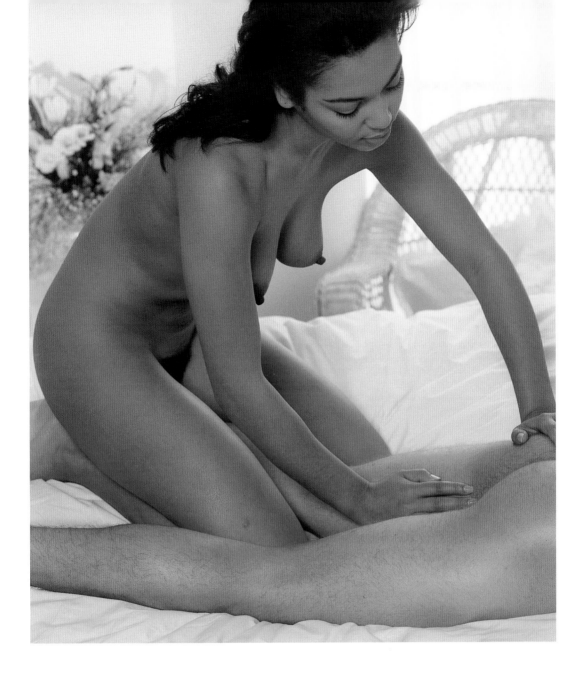

CREATE AN AIR OF INTIMACY

A massage session is to be savoured, so find a time when you won't be disturbed. Choose a warm, draught-free room and create a soft, soothing atmosphere through subdued lighting, soft music and aromatic candles. Before you begin, remove rings or other jewellery and make sure your nails are trimmed. Your partner should lie on a large towel on the bed or a carpeted floor. Always use a good-quality massage oil (known as a carrier oil), such as sunflower, grapeseed or sweet almond. Pour a little oil onto the palm of one hand, rub your hands together and then use broad, sweeping strokes to spread the oil gently over each part of your partner's body as you come to it.

KNEADING STROKES

Grasp fleshy areas between your fingers and thumbs and gently squeeze, as though you are kneading dough.

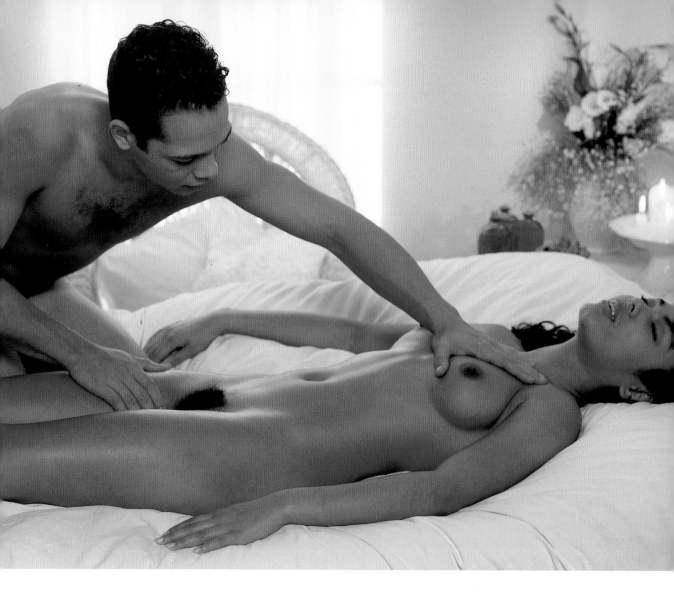

SLOW BUILD-UP

Tempting though it is to have a naked, compliant body at your fingertips, avoid the most sexually sensitive areas – at least at first. The aim is to achieve a leisurely build-up to arousal, stimulating erogenous zones only as your partner's passion mounts. Start by massaging the shoulders and back, and then work down to the buttocks and the backs of the legs. Ask your partner to turn over, and then massage the arms, torso, chest, abdomen and the front of the legs, finishing at the feet.

AROMATHERAPY OILS

To make the massage even more magical, pour the massage oil into a small bowl and add a few drops of an aromatherapy essential oil (available from pharmacies and healthfood stores). These oils are highly concentrated so they should never be used neat and the most sensitive

USE VARIETY

Vary your strokes, sometimes describing small, circular movements with your thumbs, at other times stroking your partner with feather-light touches of your fingertips.

EXPLORE

OPPOSITE: *Discover new areas of sensitivity, such as the nape of the neck, the backs of the knees or the feet.*

areas of the body are best avoided. Lavender, rosewood and geranium oils all have calming effects; sweet marjoram is good for soothing tired muscles and sandalwood oil is both relaxing and has aphrodisiac properties.

tip

For a less messy massage, don't use oil. Instead, sprinkle talcum powder over the areas you're going to work on.

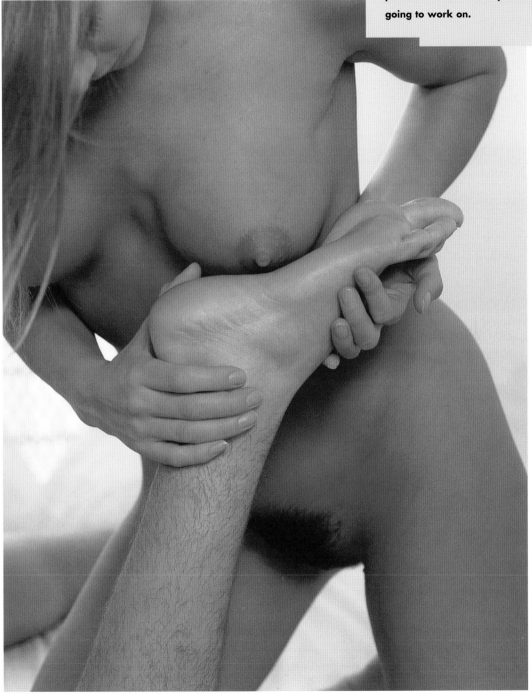

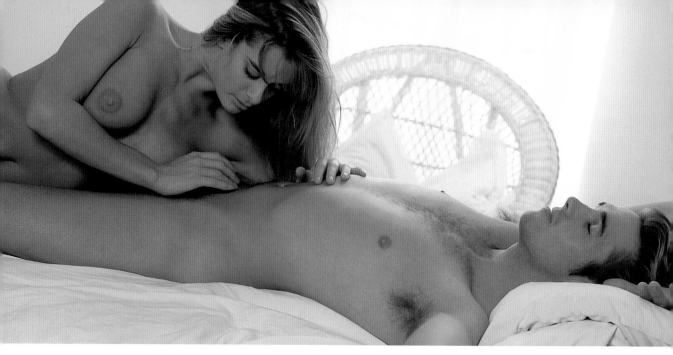

BE GUIDED

Let your partner be your guide and say what is best for him or her, applying more pressure or less as he or she requests it.

KEEP IN TOUCH

Always keep one hand on your partner, even when you are adding more oil. Simply pour the oil over the back of the hand that is in contact with your lover and use the other hand to rub it onto his or her body.

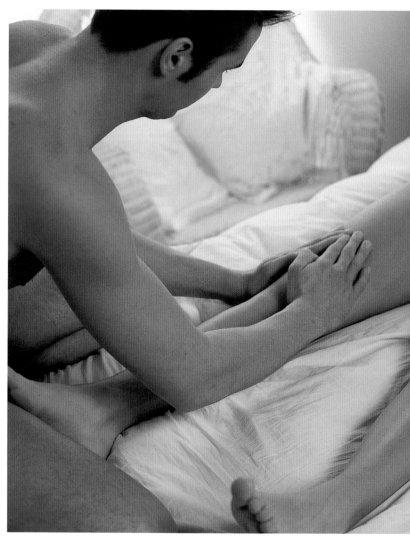

warning

If you're pregnant, avoid using essential oils or ask a qualified aromatherapist to recommend oils you can use with safety.

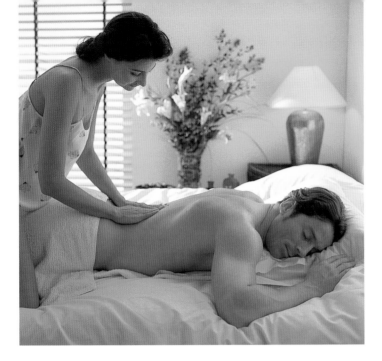

RELIEVING STRESS

Give a massage whenever your partner is too stressed, anxious or tired for lovemaking. It offers an emotionally satisfying alternative to sex, promoting a sense of trust and intimacy that will enhance your relationship.

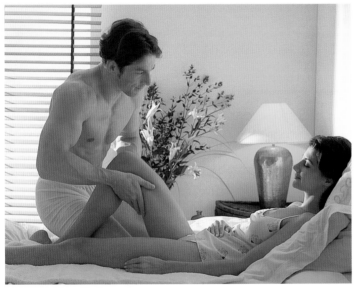

EASING TENSION

Over fleshy areas, use squeezing or kneading movements, especially where you feel tension, such as knotted muscles. But avoid being too rough as the aim is for a soothing and gently arousing massage.

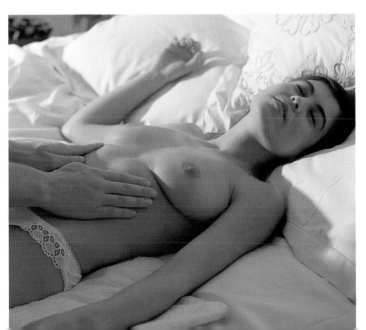

VARY THE PRESSURE

As you massage each area, begin with a light touch, moulding your hands to the contours of your partner's body, and slowly increase the pressure. Return to light pressure before sliding on to the next part of the body.

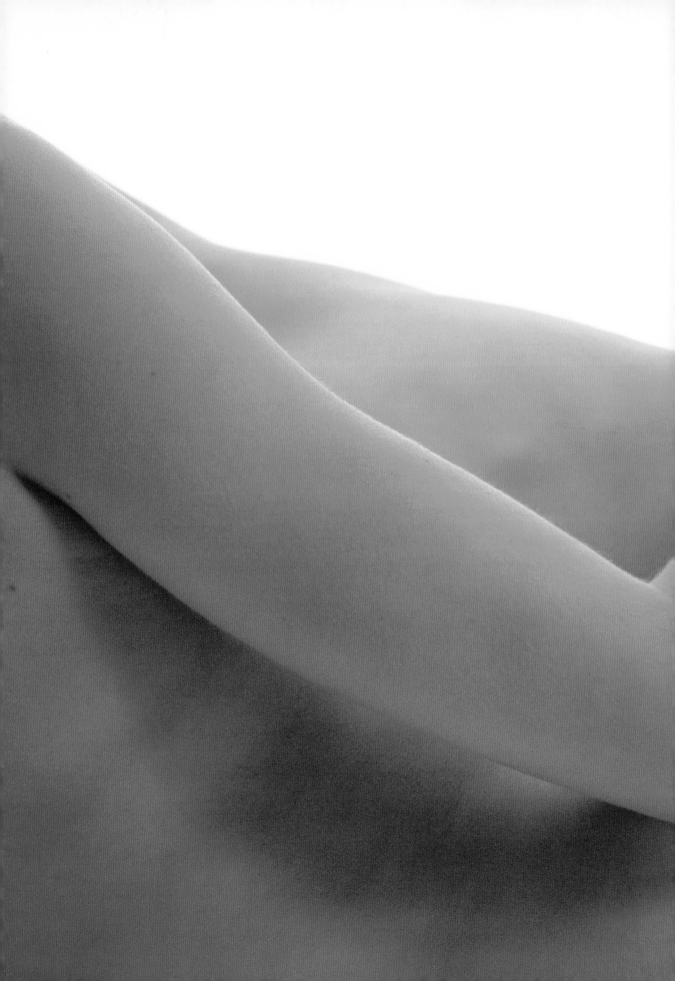

THE
FUN OF
FOREPLAY

FOREPLAY IS IMPORTANT, SO COUPLES SHOULD ALWAYS MAKE TIME FOR IT, ESPECIALLY

AS MOST WOMEN FEEL SEXUALLY FULFILLED ONLY AFTER A LONG, SLOW BUILD-UP. THE

TIME COUPLES SPEND IN FOREPLAY CAN HEIGHTEN THEIR PLEASURE AND STRENGTHEN

THE BONDS OF LOVE AND FRIENDSHIP BETWEEN THEM.

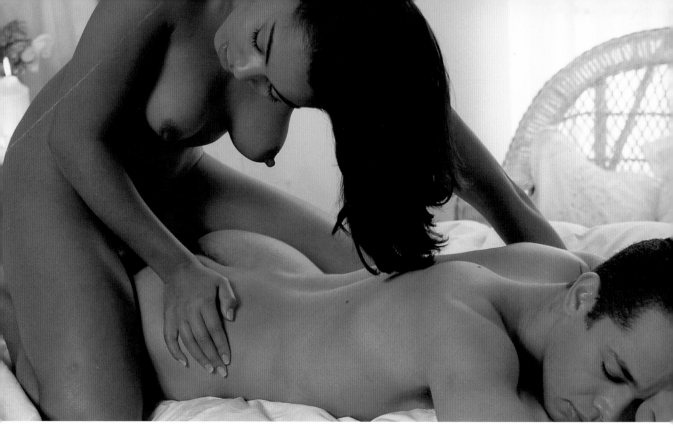

SENSITIVE STIMULATION

Many women say their sexual partners never take time to find out what turns them on but foreplay offers the ideal opportunity. It involves kissing, caressing, touching and stroking a partner in ways he or she finds especially arousing. This is a good time to discover a lover's most sensitive erogenous zones – and the best way to stimulate them. A woman should make it clear what she likes, and doesn't like, and encourage her partner to experiment. By listening and responding to his partner's needs, a man will find that sex is enhanced for both of them. It also shows his partner that he really enjoys the look and feel of her body and is keen to make their lovemaking last.

TICKLE AND TANTALIZE

Let your fingers touch, stroke and squeeze, and your lips and tongue lick and suck your lover. Use your nose, breasts and toes to tickle and tease. Try stroking your partner with your hair, a feather, a piece of silk or rub on some oil to heighten the sensation.

NIBBLING

Playful biting and nibbling can be highly arousing, but you should always be gentle and try not to leave marks. Avoid the most sensitive areas, such as the nipples, clitoris, labia, penis orscrotum (or make sure you cover your teeth with your lips).

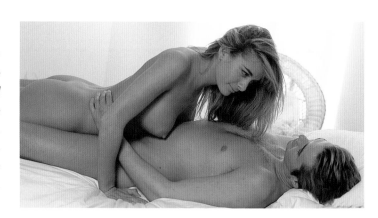

THE PLEASURE PRINCIPLE

Try to please – and tantalize – your partner, using whatever ideas your fertile imagination can dream up. The aim is to build up desire and anticipation slowly so, initially, avoid the genital area. A woman's body is covered with erogenous zones, any one of which may respond to a teasing hand. While a man's body is more limited in this respect, he will still enjoy a woman's touch on his chest, back, buttocks and, especially, the perineum. Although foreplay is usually a preliminary to sex, it doesn't have to lead to full intercourse. It is also a wonderful way for a couple to relax and be intimate with one another without feeling under any pressure to fulfil a 'sexual goal'.

TOUCH AND TEASE

BELOW LEFT: *Explore your partner's body, seeking out new pleasure zones that he or she never knew existed. For instance, lavish your attention on the ears, neck, stomach, thighs, backs of the knees and calves, before moving on to the buttocks, breasts, nipples and inner thighs.*

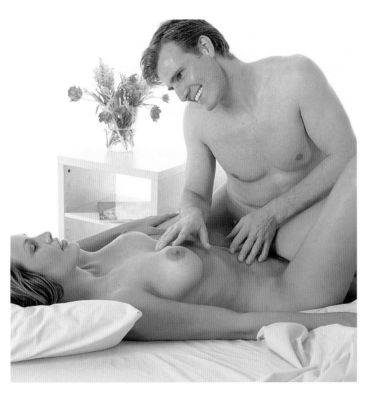

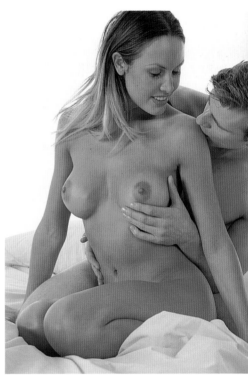

SELF-PLEASURING

Men are often accused of a lack of subtlety or finesse in the way they touch a woman's body, while many men say women are not firm enough. A good way to find out how hard your partner likes to be touched is to watch them as they pleasure themselves. As well as being informative, it can be highly arousing to watch a lover rub, stroke and caress his or her own body and it won't be long before you'll want to join in. From self-pleasuring, you can caress and stroke each other's body until you climax or switch to another position for lovemaking.

TENDER TOUCH

ABOVE: *Guide your partner to those areas you enjoy being touched and encourage him with words and sounds to show how much he is arousing you.*

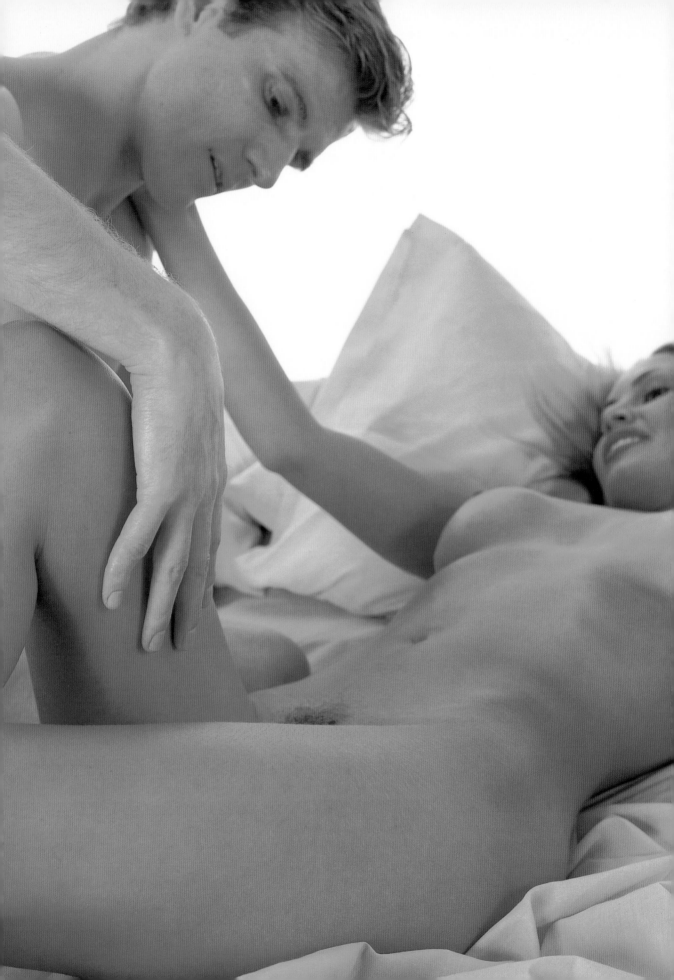

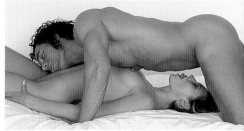

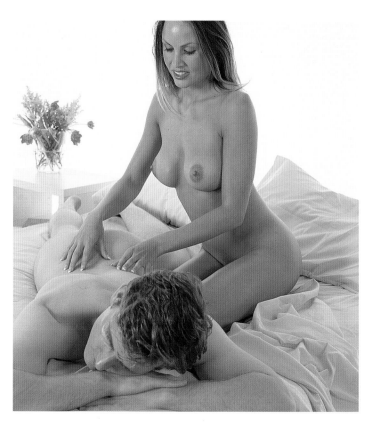

VOYAGE OF EXPLORATION

LEFT: *For men, the loving contact of petting helps to broaden their experience of sex and trains them to control and pace their sexual feelings.*

ENJOYING EACH OTHER

ABOVE: *Foreplay is the ideal time to explore different sensations before the urgency of your passion takes over. The skin of the abdomen is very sensitive and responds to the delicate touch of the tongue.*

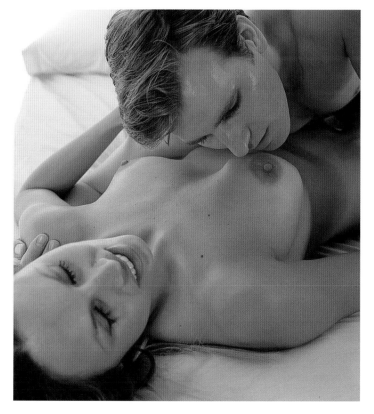

THE PLEASURE OF PETTING

LEFT AND OPPOSITE: *Women usually need emotional – as well as physical – stimulation, so petting is important. It is a way for couples to show mutual love, trust and enjoyment of each other's body through tender touching.*

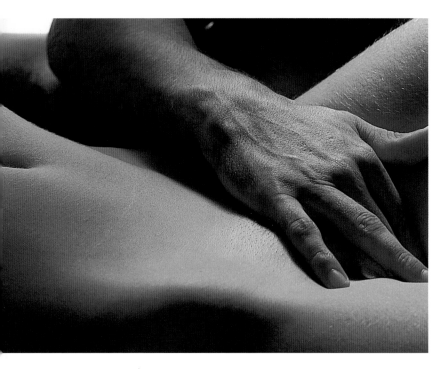

EXPERT TOUCH

Once you've seen how your partner likes to be stimulated, take over to show them what you have learnt. Start slowly and prolong the pleasure as long as possible.

MUTUAL MASTURBATION

RIGHT: Pleasuring each other provides shared moments of intimacy that help you to bond as a couple and take the relationship to a deeper level.

masturbating her

When masturbating a woman, try to vary your pressure and movement and the parts of her genitals you're stimulating.

Be guided by your partner, altering the degree of stimulation to match her responses. For example:

- Squeeze the outer labia gently between finger and thumb, and then slowly rub them up and down.

- Apply finger or palm pressure to the pubic mound and clitoral area, and then rub, alternating up and down and circular motions.

- When your partner's vagina is well-lubricated, insert a finger into the opening and move it gently in and out, while pressing the knuckles of your other fingers against her clitoral area.

- Insert a finger into her vagina and rub its front wall (try to find her G-spot, page 11), at the same time rubbing the clitoral area with your thumb or palm, or try fingering her anus lightly.

- Maintain the same pace and movement as she climaxes (she will tense up and you may feel her vagina contract rhythmically) and continue until she relaxes, indicating that her orgasm is over.

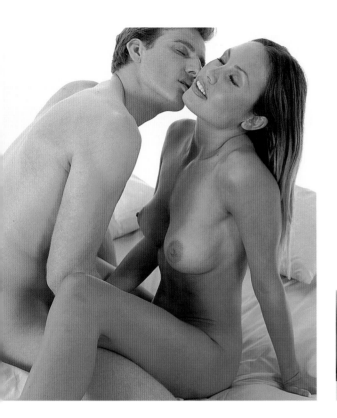

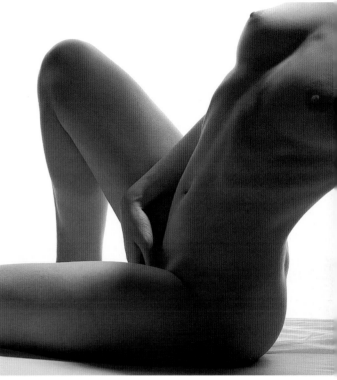

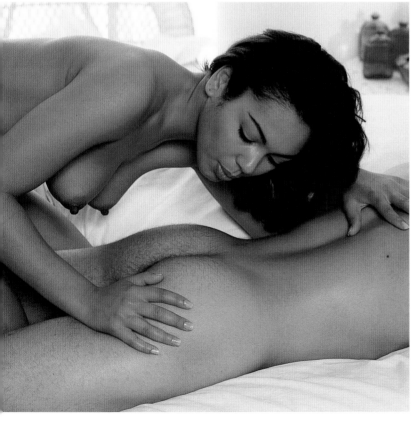

PLEASURING HERSELF

Pleasure yourself to show your partner how you like to be stimulated. It will be a turn-on for him and also helps to release any inhibitions.

HOT AIR

If you moisten your lover's skin with your tongue and gently blow across it, you can create an electrifying experience that can drive them wild.

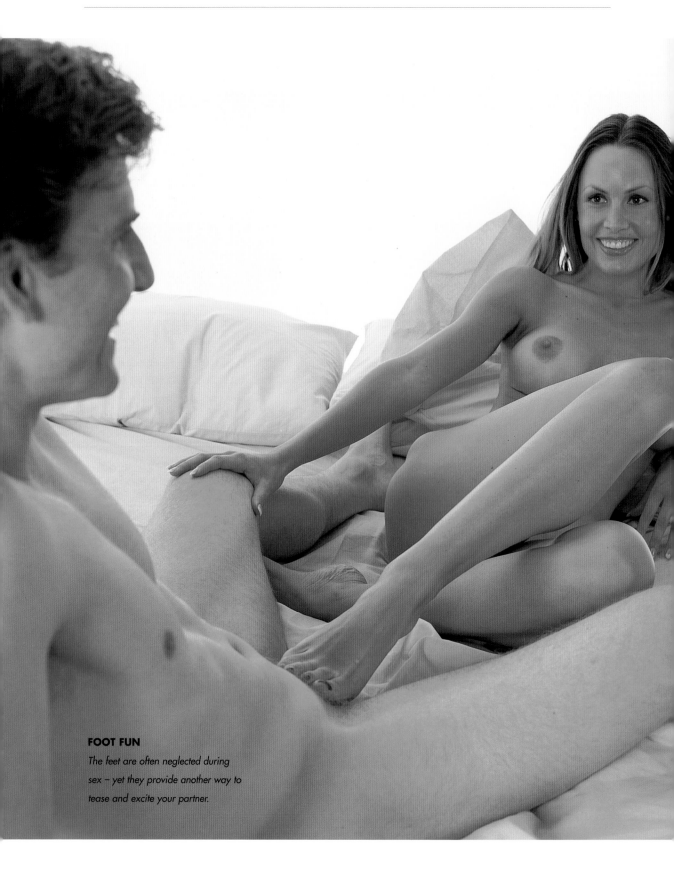

FOOT FUN

The feet are often neglected during sex – yet they provide another way to tease and excite your partner.

BREAST FRIENDS

Be inventive in the way you use your body to arouse a lover. For example, squeeze your partner's penis between your breasts as you plant moist kisses on his belly.

PLEASURING HIMSELF

For women, too, the sight of a partner pleasuring himself can be powerfully arousing, as well as instructive.

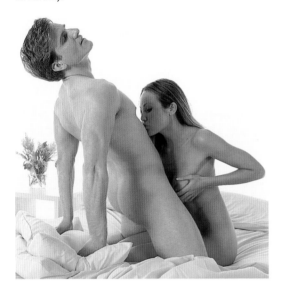

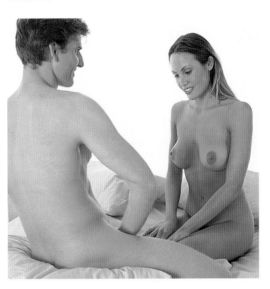

masturbating him

Your partner will enjoy being stimulated by you, but he may want to guide your hand with his, at least initially, to show how he wants you to do it. Experiment with different techniques, for example:

- Using thumb and forefinger, grip his penis just under the head and rub up and down while fondling his testicles with your other hand and gently squeezing them.

- Squeeze the top of the shaft and rub a finger over the frenulum.

- If he is uncircumcized, rub and squeeze the foreskin over the glans. And if he has been circumcized, gently rub over and around the glans.

- With thumb and forefinger, grip the shaft. Rub up and down, using long, slow strokes initially. Steadily increase speed and pressure. To increase stimulation, rub close to the head of the penis. As he climaxes, the glans becomes very sensitive so you may need to rub closer to the base until he finishes ejaculating.

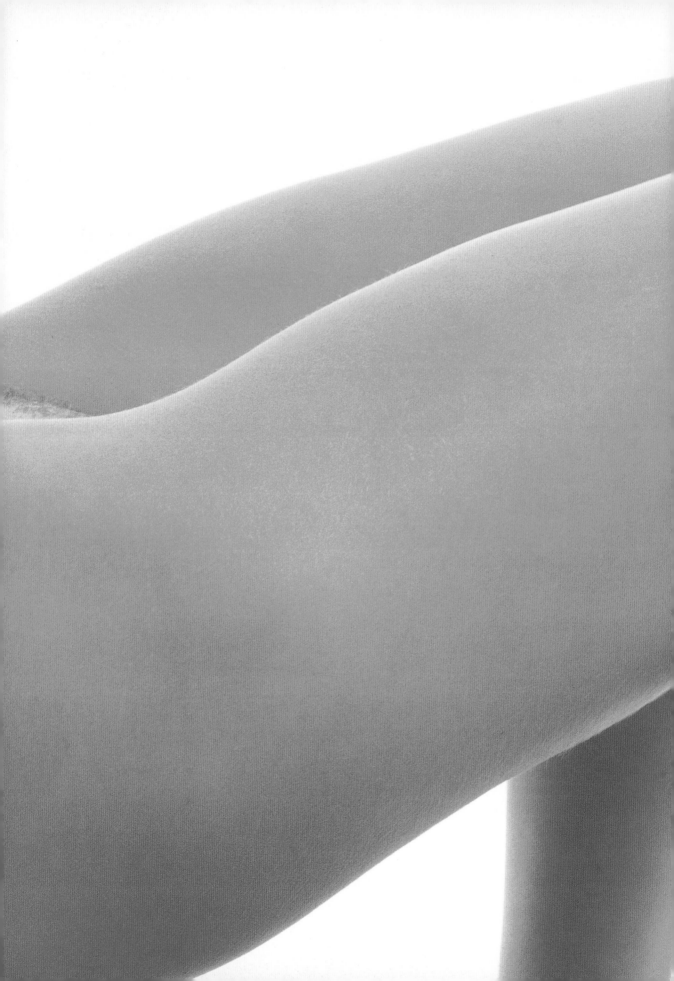

7 PAYING LIP SERVICE

FOR MANY COUPLES, ORAL SEX – USING YOUR MOUTH AND TONGUE TO STIMULATE YOUR PARTNER'S GENITALS – IS THE ULTIMATE SEXUAL EXPERIENCE. THE GIVER ENJOYS THE EROTIC SIGHT, FEEL AND SCENT OF THEIR PARTNER'S SEXUAL ORGANS WHILE THE RECEIVER SIMPLY LIES BACK AND IS TRANSPORTED TO PARADISE.

ORAL SEX FOR HER

Oral sex performed on a woman is called 'cunnilingus', taken from the Latin words for 'vulva' and 'licking'. It offers the most intimate of sexual delights and, with patience and sensitivity, is powerfully arousing; many women easily achieve multiple orgasms this way. For a man, performing oral sex can be almost as erotic as receiving it, so he should take his time. With the woman's thighs spread comfortably wide, her vulva is easily accessible to his lips and tongue. As this is the most sensitive part of his partner's body, the man should first stimulate other areas, for example, kissing and licking the woman's inner thighs and lower abdomen before approaching her vulva.

MOUTH MAGIC

The easiest position for cunnilingus is for the woman to lie back on the bed with her parted legs over the edge. The man then kneels down in front of her.

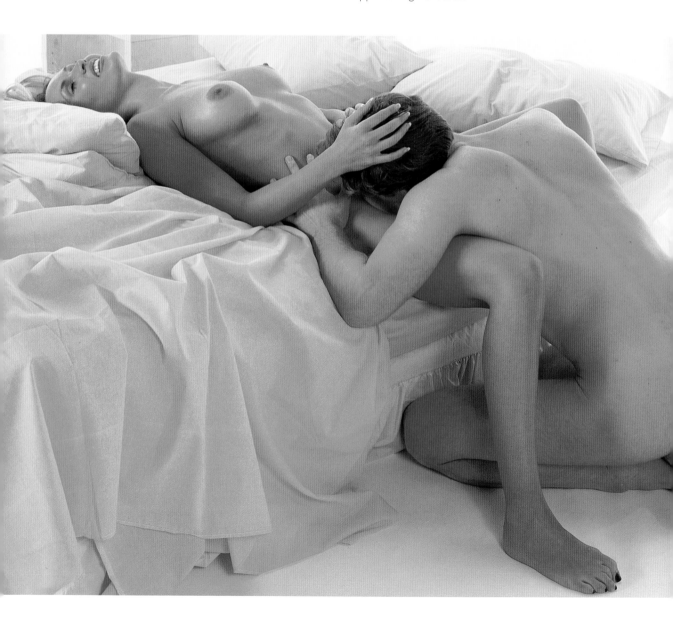

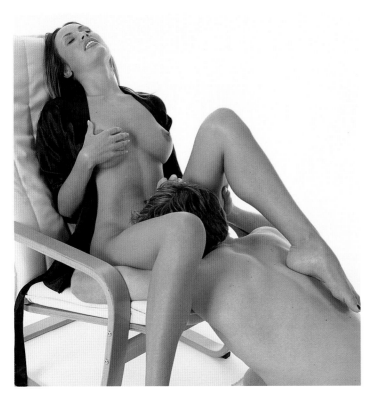

CHAIR DELIGHT

For spontaneous oral sex, clothed or unclothed, the woman can sit in a chair with her thighs spread wide while the man kneels to place his head between them.

CROUCHING CLIMAX

Many women like to squat over their partner's face and slowly bring their vulva into close proximity with his mouth.

BUILD THE TENSION

Through gentle, teasing movements the man can build the sexual tension until his partner thinks she's going to explode. He can then gently part her pubic hair with his fingers and pause to enjoy the sight. By partly covering his teeth with his lips, he can gently nibble on the outer labia. Then, with his head deep between her thighs, he can lick upward, using long tongue strokes, and keeping his actions firm, but gentle. His tongue is a flexible device for exploring her vagina, thrusting it in as deep as he can reach and savouring her love juices. He should experiment with different actions, varying his movements, perhaps nuzzling and then sucking, or following slow, teasing licks with more rapid, forceful ones. His partner may also enjoy being simultaneously fingered. The man should follow his partner's lead and be guided by her, easing off if he gets too rough, or increasing the pace to match her arousal.

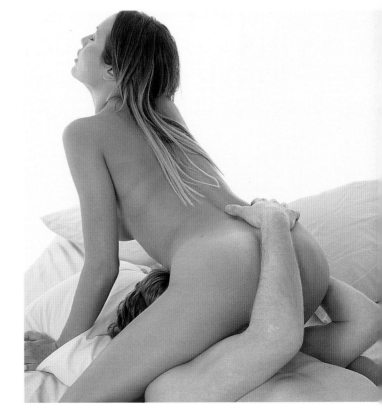

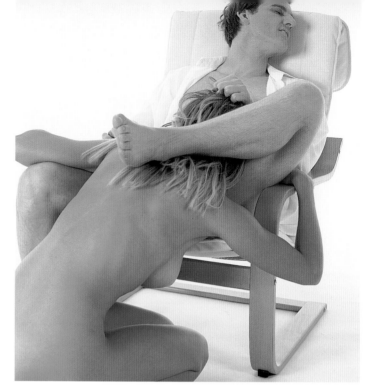

SEAT OF PLEASURE

Some men enjoy oral sex most when sitting in a chair, while their partner kneels before them.

SHE'S IN CHARGE

OPPOSITE: *When performing fellatio, a woman has most control when her partner lies on his back, while she lies over him and takes his penis in her mouth.*

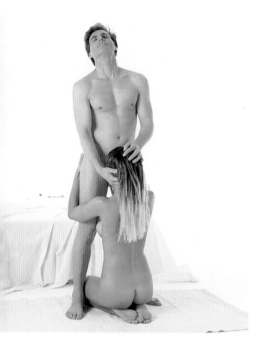

FREE-STANDING FUN

Another fellatio position is for the man to stand up, with the woman kneeling in front of him, so that his erect penis is level with her face.

ORAL SEX FOR HIM

When performed on a man, oral sex is called 'fellatio', from the Latin for 'sucking', and is regarded by many as the greatest sexual favour a woman can bestow. Emotionally, it can be highly gratifying to have a woman pay such close attention to a man. Fellatio is so arousing that a man may ejaculate too soon, before he's had a chance to enjoy the experience fully, so it is often reserved for foreplay or to re-arouse a flaccid penis after he has previously ejaculated.

Sexual tools

A woman's versatile mouth and tongue make great sexual tools, being able to caress areas of the man's penis and testicles that could not be stimulated so powerfully in other ways. But she needn't limit herself to his sexual organs. To increase the sexual tension, she could work from his neck to his chest before slowly making her way to his navel. Then she can caress his thighs before reaching his genitals. At first, a woman may need to grip her partner's penis with her fingers, but with practice, she'll be able to use her mouth alone and give him extra pleasure by simultaneously stroking other parts of his body.

All parts of a man's genitals are highly sensitive, but he will find it especially arousing if his partner uses her lips and tongue to stimulate the sensitive little frenulum and the delicate skin of the scrotum. The woman may start by licking the shaft of his penis with delicate, upward strokes and then flick her tongue lightly from side to side. She can swirl

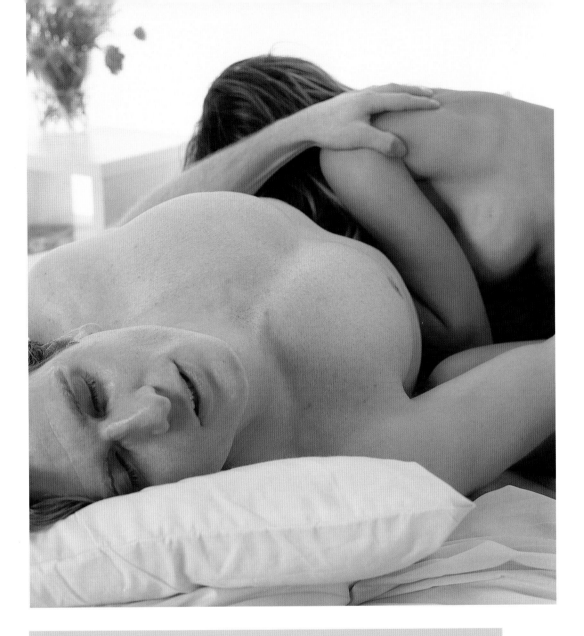

sexual hygiene

Sexual hygiene is important, especially for uncircumcized men, who must take care to prevent a build-up of an oily secretion called 'smegma' under the foreskin. Wash the genitals and anal area with soap or other cleanser, but avoid highly-fragranced soaps and deodorants. These mask the natural scents that men and women find erotic and often have an unpleasant chemical taste that can put partners off oral sex. Cunnilingus is more pleasant for the woman when the man is smoothly-shaven. Remember, too, that cold sores on or around the mouth can be transmitted and may cause genital herpes; also garlic or spicy breath is fine if you have both eaten the same kind of food!

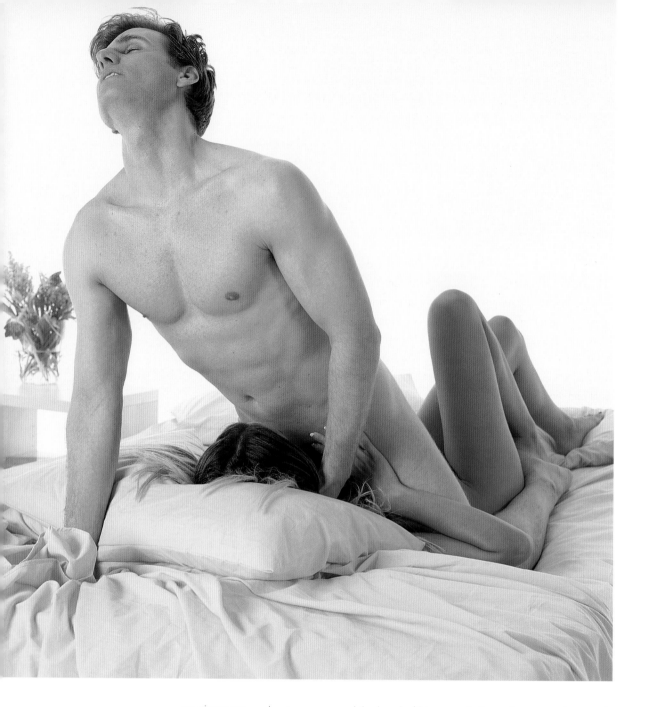

IN CONTROL

A man may like to control the action by kneeling over his partner, supporting his weight on his arms and knees, while she lies on her back. The woman has little control in this position, however, so the man must take care not to thrust too deeply.

her tongue around the head of his penis, before taking it into her mouth and sucking it gently, while moving her mouth up and down.

Once his penis is in her mouth, the woman's partner can place his hands on her head to guide her rhythm without being too forceful while respecting her right to withdraw at any time. She'll be able to tell when he's close to climaxing through changes in his breathing, tension in his thighs and abdomen, and the increasing hardness of his penis. Many women like to continue fellatio until their partner ejaculates: semen is harmless (and contains sugar, so it's nutritious, too!) and it can be safely swallowed (but see Safer Sex, page 123). But if she prefers, a woman can bring the man to orgasm by hand, or, for example, by rubbing his penis between her breasts (page 55).

Soixante-neuf ('69')

Mutual oral sex is also known as 'soixante-neuf', which is French for '69' and describes the 'top-to-tail' position of the man and woman. This position is so erotic that men may find it difficult to prevent themselves from ejaculating too soon. Therefore, couples often use soixante-neuf just to heighten sexual arousal, and then switch to another position. It is difficult to perform oral sex with care and sensitivity when you're close to orgasm yourself (it's not unknown for a woman to bite her partner's penis at the critical moment!), so consider taking turns. As a man gets aroused more easily than a woman, it is best if he stimulates her first. His partner may enjoy several orgasms, and be ready for more, before it is his turn to be pleasured. The woman can keep her mouth actions light and teasing to prolong his enjoyment.

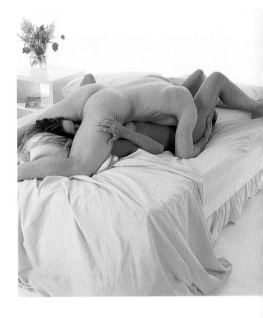

SOIXANTE-NEUF

It is important to find a position for soixante-neuf that is comfortable for both of you. In the standard position, either the man or woman can be on top, but whoever is below is likely to get a stiff neck.

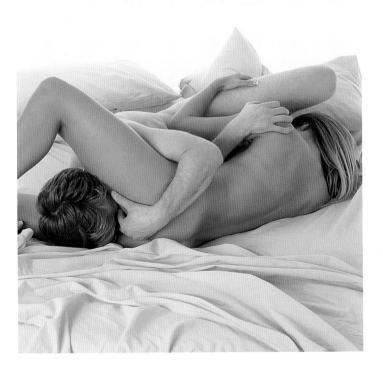

PILLOW PARTNERS

A more relaxed position for soixante-neuf is to lie side by side, with the lower leg drawn up as a pillow to support the partner's head. The man is then free to kiss and lick his partner's vulva while she sucks his penis.

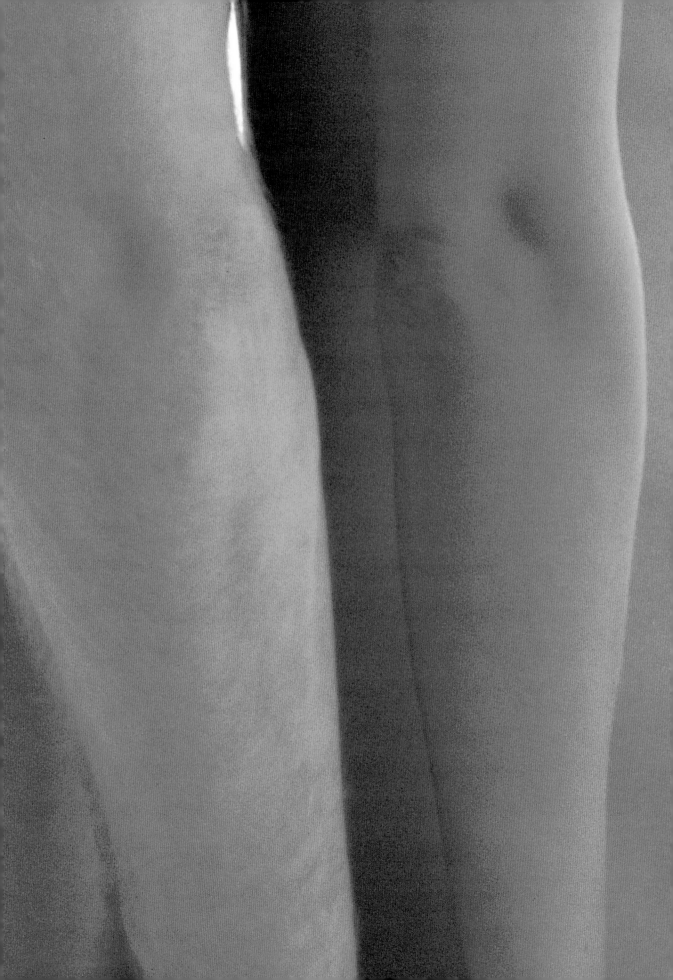

FLEXIBLE FRIENDS

MANY COUPLES REGARD PENETRATIVE SEX AS THE ULTIMATE FORM OF SEXUAL

EXPRESSION. RIGHTLY OR WRONGLY, THEY THINK ORGASMS ACHIEVED BY PENILE

STIMULATION OF THE VAGINA HAVE A VALUE AND INTENSITY LACKING IN OTHER

POSITIONS. FORTUNATELY, THE FLEXIBLE HUMAN FRAME ALLOWS AN AMAZING

VARIETY OF WAYS TO HELP THEM ACHIEVE THIS.

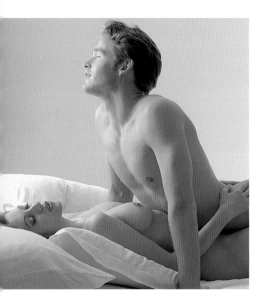

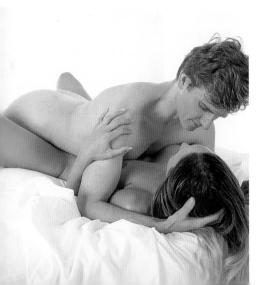

MAN ON TOP

The man-on-top or 'missionary' position is the standard one for penetrative sex. The man lies on top of his partner with his body between her parted thighs. He takes his weight on his hands or elbows and pushes his penis into her vagina, hopefully bringing them both to orgasm through rhythmic thrusts of his pelvis. Man-on-top positions are popular because they allow full eye contact and passionate kissing. However, the woman has a mainly passive role and the man's penis doesn't strongly stimulate some of the most sensitive areas of her genitals, so she may need extra stimulation. Her partner should ensure she is already highly aroused before settling into this position. Then, by supporting himself on one arm, he can keep a hand free to caress her body and help her to climax.

WOMAN ON TOP

For a female, the woman-on-top position is often the best way to get an orgasm through penetrative sex because she can decide on the angle and pace at which the man's penis stimulates her vagina. In particular, it offers more effective stimulation of the G-spot on the front wall of the vagina (see page 11). With the man almost helpless beneath her, she takes control, choosing the moment to lower herself onto him and to guide his penis into herself with her hand.

By varying her movements she can enhance her satisfaction, and can easily stroke her clitoris to bring herself to orgasm. For the man, too, this is a highly enjoyable position. All he has to do is lie back while she takes charge, slowing her pace deliciously to prolong the pleasure. As his partner is doing all the work, the man is free to enjoy her facial expressions, feel her breasts and stroke her thighs.

SIDE BY SIDE

Side by side is the most relaxed and loving position, ideal for slow, intimate sex. Neither partner dominates as they lie, entwined, making love. Women like the intimate eye contact, the feeling of being secure and loved, and the fact that they're in equal control of the pace and depth of penetration. Many men like it because the restricted movement helps them to prolong sex. The vagina is more constricted than in other positions, which can increase the friction, and hence the stimulation, for both partners. Lying side by side, a man may find it difficult to caress his partner's breasts and vulva. Instead, he can concentrate on often-neglected areas of her body, such as her spine, hips and buttocks. By alternating periods of thrusting with moments spent in a loving embrace, caressing each other's body, the couple can enhance the loving element as well as prolonging sex. They can choose to stay in this position or easily switch to the man- or woman-on-top position.

REAR ENTRY

Rear entry is a versatile position that can be performed sitting, standing, kneeling, bending, side by side or with the woman on top. For the man, it allows greater depth of penetration and for the woman, it offers direct contact with the back wall of her vagina and her perineum and buttocks. To increase stimulation, the woman can raise her buttocks and push back with her pelvis in time with the man's thrusts. The man can reach round to stroke his partner's breasts, pubic mound and clitoris to increase her arousal – or simply enjoy the feel of her.

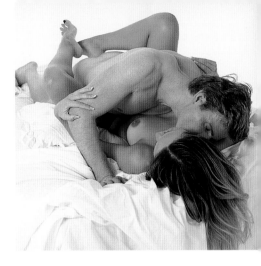

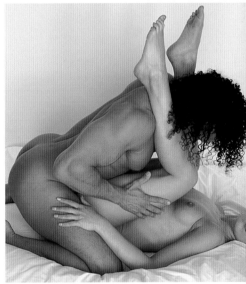

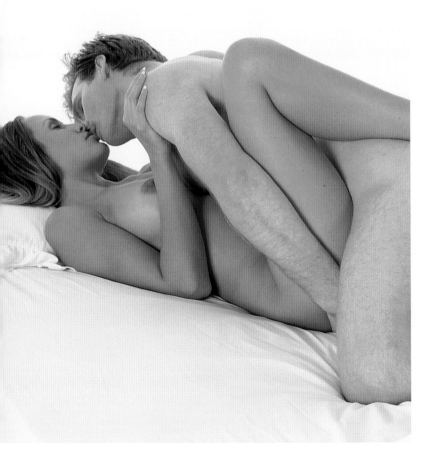

MATRIMONIAL

TOP: *By wrapping her legs around the man's waist the woman has some control over his thrusting movements and can direct his penis to where she feels it will do her most good.*

BURGUNDIAN

ABOVE: *If the woman is supple enough, she can wrap her ankles around the man's neck. By bringing his knees up close he increases depth of penetration and stimulates different areas.*

FLANQUETTE

LEFT: *This is a variation of the missionary position. The man places one of his legs between the woman's and she, likewise, puts one of her legs between his. This gives her more control with added clitoral stimulation from the man's thigh.*

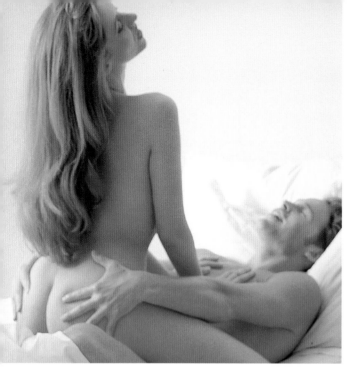
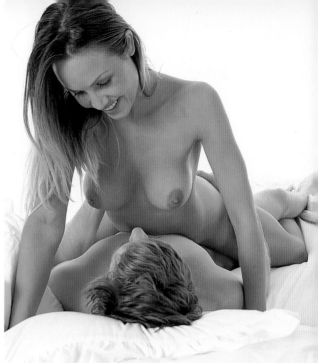

ST GEORGE

Many women like to sit astride their partner, alternating up and down movements with gentle side-to-side or back-and-forth rocking actions. This position is the most energetic for the woman, but affords her total flexibility to alter her position.

ST GEORGE (VARIATION)

By leaning further forward and flattening her body, the woman can alter the angle of entry of the man's penis and increase skin-to-skin contact and the feeling of intimacy.

REVERSE ST GEORGE

By reversing her position, so that her back is to the man, a woman can use her partner's penis to stimulate different regions of her vagina. The man can easily reach around her waist to caress her breasts and vulva.

MOTHER SUPERIOR

By lying on top of the man with her legs between his, the woman slows down the pace of lovemaking while tightening the muscles of her vagina, thereby increasing the friction of his penis inside her.

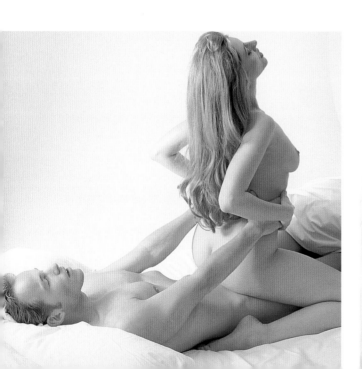
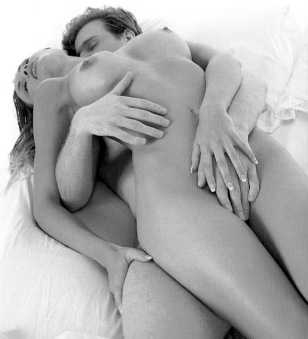

STANDARD SIDE BY SIDE

To reach the side-by-side position, the easiest way is to roll over from the missionary or woman-on-top position. The woman lifts one leg and wraps it over the man's waist while enfolding him in her arms.

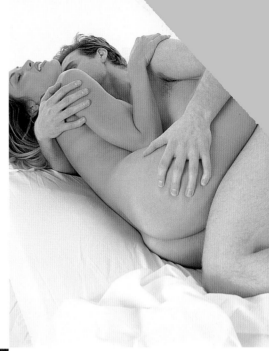

TOP-TO-TOE TITILLATION

For maximum skin-to-skin contact, the women can lie along the top of her man, moving slowly backward and forward to rub her clitoris against him. She can press down on his feet for extra impetus.

RAISED SIDE BY SIDE

The freedom of movement side by side affords lets either partner change leg position to alter the angle of penetration and allows the couple to switch to another sexual position with ease.

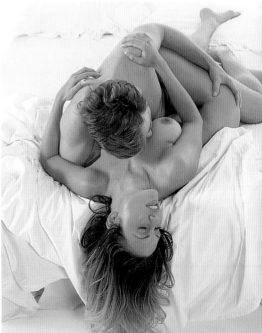

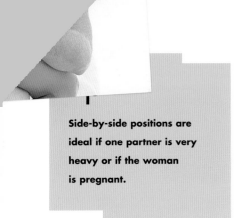

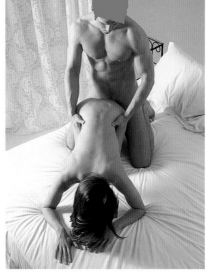

Side-by-side positions are ideal if one partner is very heavy or if the woman is pregnant.

DOGGY FASHION

This is the best-known position for rear entry, with the woman kneeling on the bed, taking her weight on her elbows, while the man kneels behind her, with his legs between or behind hers.

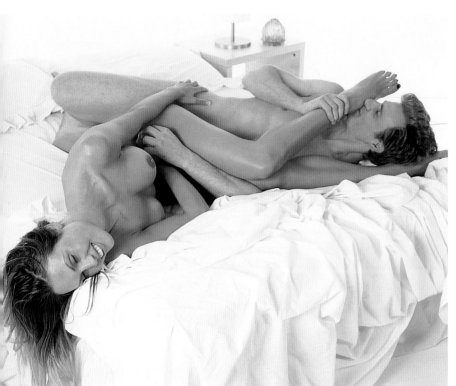

SIDE BURGUNDIAN

If the woman wraps her legs around her partner's neck while they remain in the side-by-side position, the man can achieve much deeper penetration. To enhance the stimulation, they can rock their bodies in synchrony, starting slowly and steadily increasing the pace as their arousal grows.

CROUPADE

This is an intensely erotic form of rear-entry sex, in which the woman takes her weight on her hands and keeps her knees slightly bent. The man remains standing and enters her from behind. (It is not advisable for women with a weak back and should only be attempted on firm flooring!)

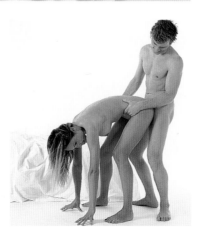

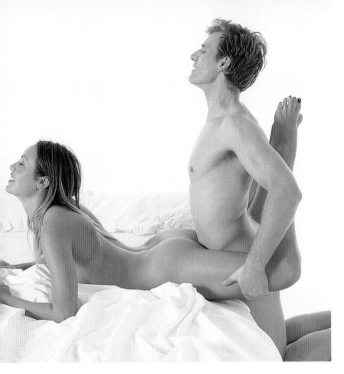

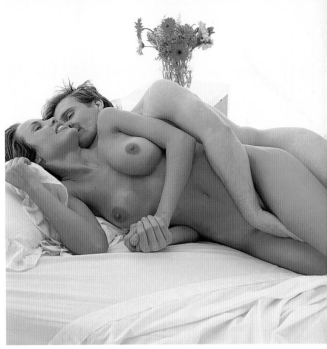

SUPPORTED CROUPADE

If the woman wants more support, she can kneel on the floor and rest her upper body or elbows on a chair or bed. The man kneels or remains standing and can lift his partner's legs to change the angle of entry.

SPOONS

A gentle and relaxed rear-entry position. The couple lie on their sides and the man enters his partner from behind. Like the side-by-side position, it provides a slow and tender form of lovemaking which is good in pregnancy or when you're tired.

SERVANTE D'AMOUR

In this position, the woman kneels on the bed, supporting herself on her elbows with her hands clasped behind her neck. The man kneels behind her and supports himself with his hands on her upper back. By hooking her legs around his, she can pull him tightly toward her.

CUISSADE

This is a half rear-, half side-entry position with the woman partly turned toward her partner. She keeps one leg between those of her partner and the other one drawn up across her abdomen.

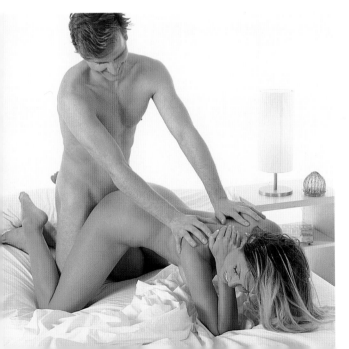

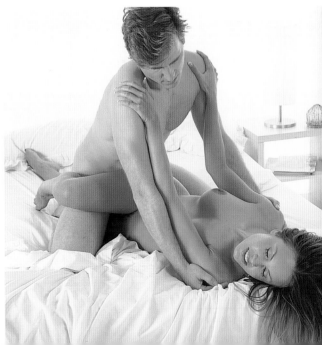

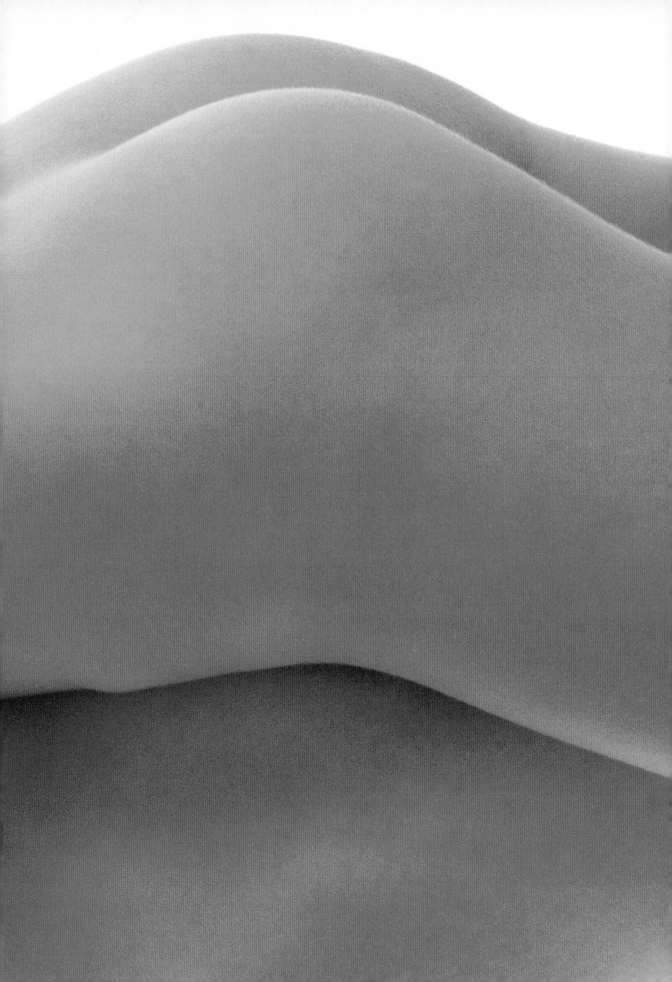

'It doesn't matter what you do in the bedroom as long as you don't do it in the street and frighten the horses.'

MRS PATRICK CAMPBELL

A DASH OF SPICE

VARIETY IS THE SPICE OF A HEALTHY SEX LIFE. TALKING ABOUT, AND EXPERIMENTING

WITH, DIFFERENT POSITIONS AND MOVEMENTS CAN ENCOURAGE COMMUNICATION

BETWEEN PARTNERS AND ADD SOME FUN AND SPARKLE TO A RELATIONSHIP.

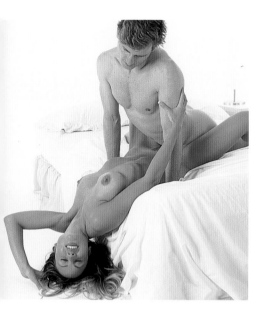

ADVENTUROUS SEX

Trying different sexual positions can enhance a relationship as it shows that both partners care enough to be inventive and to find new ways to please each other. The more adventurous positions can add playfulness and excitement to sex, and produce novel pelvic sensations that couldn't be achieved in other ways. If a position gives a pleasurable feeling, a man or woman should share this fact with their partner. Bear in mind, though, that some positions may cause injury unless performed correctly and so shouldn't be attempted unless both partners feel confident that they're not taking risks. The man in particular should also feel strong enough to cope with them and they should both be fairly supple.

INVERSION

For a new experience, inversion can create mind-blowing orgasms for the woman. In the Australian position, the woman lies over the edge of the bed with her head practically touching the floor as her partner makes love to her. The rush of blood can greatly intensify the moment of climax for her. For the athletic, the 'Wheelbarrow' allows the man to raise the woman's legs as she walks on her hands, head down, along the floor. For a slightly easier version, the woman can support herself on her elbows on the bed.

AUSTRALIAN

This position needs great care and is only for the fit and healthy, but well worth the effort. It causes a rush of blood to the head that can really enhance the sexual high. The woman lies on the edge of the bed with her head touching the floor, supporting herself with her hands.

QUICKIE SEX

For raw, animal passion, when you and your partner are too aroused to wait a moment longer, you can't beat quickie sex. As lust overwhelms you, there's just enough time to clear a space on a nearby table as, tearing at each other's clothes, you give in to your desires and re-enact the famous movie scene in *The Postman Only Rings Twice*. Sometimes there isn't even a table close by. No problem. Sex standing up, perhaps leaning up against a wall or door (check it's firmly shut first!) is an unforgettable experience. And if the woman grips her partner's waist with her legs and leans back, she can experience a combination of inverted and quickie sex at the same time.

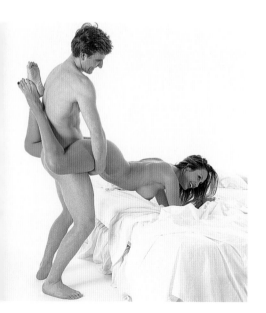

WHEELBARROW

In this version of the wheelbarrow, the woman supports her upper body on the bed while her partner stands upright between her legs. By gripping her thighs, he can raise her legs to change the angle of entry.

PASSION MOUNTS ...

The most fun you can have standing up ... For quickie sex, clothed or naked, the couple hold each other tightly as they plant breathless kisses on each other's eager faces.

... DRAWING HIM IN

Slowly, the woman raises one leg and wraps it around her partner, drawing her body toward him. He supports her lower back as he enters her.

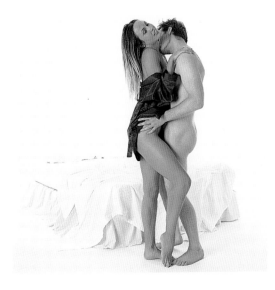

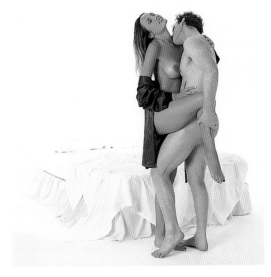

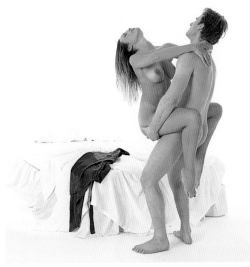

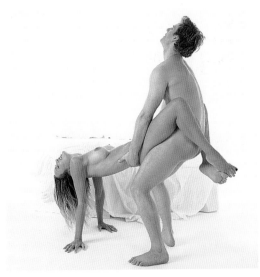

... HOLD ON TIGHT

As the man holds his partner firmly, she raises her other leg and grips him tightly. With her arms wrapped around his neck, he can begin his pelvic thrusts while she pulls herself against him. For extra support, she can lean back against a wall or closed door.

STANDING OVATION!

For an agile couple, this advanced position adds a new dimension. By leaning right back so that her head is upside down, the woman can support herself on her hands while her partner holds her firmly. The rush of blood to her head adds to the thrill.

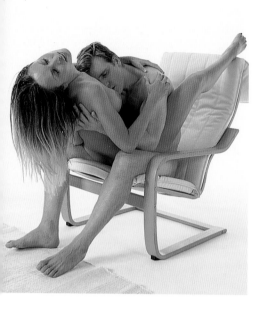

CHAIR SEX

Sex in a chair, with the woman sitting astride her partner, offers several benefits. Many couples like the fact that a hard chair allows firmer support than a soft mattress and the woman can control the depth and pace of penetration as she rocks her pelvis to and fro. Chair sex allows moments of spontaneous sex, since the woman can take the initiative whenever she feels powerfully aroused by climbing aboard her partner. From a session of heavy petting, with just a small adjustment of clothing, a couple can soon be in the throws of sexual ecstasy.

For slow and adventurous sex, make love in an armchair. With the man seated and the woman sitting in his lap with her legs around his she can dictate the depth and the rate of penetration to suit her needs as well as her partner's. In this position, the man has little to do other than use his hands and mouth to best effect on his partner's breasts, neck and shoulders.

ARMCHAIR SEX

ABOVE: *For spontaneous passion, an armchair provides limitless possibilities. With her partner seated, the women can climb into his lap and wrap her legs around his waist. If the man supports her back, she can lean back so her hands are on the floor and her head is upside down.*

SLAV POSITION

BELOW: *The woman lies on her back on the edge of the bed. Her partner stands by the bed and enters her, while gripping her ankles to hold them over her head. The man can penetrate his partner very deeply, so he must take care not to push too far or too hard.*

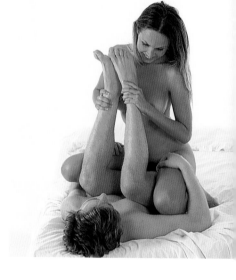

REVERSE SLAV

A woman can experience the same feeling of domination by reversing the roles. Her partner lies on his back with his knees drawn up and his legs raised. The woman then squats above him with his feet against her shoulders. (In this position she has almost total control).

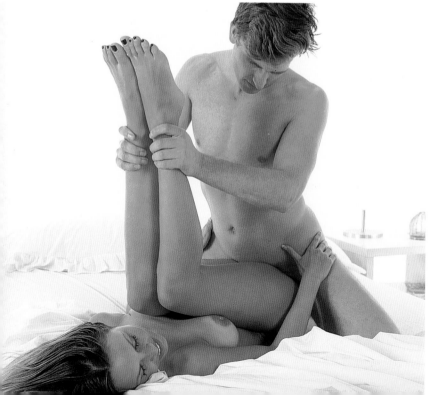

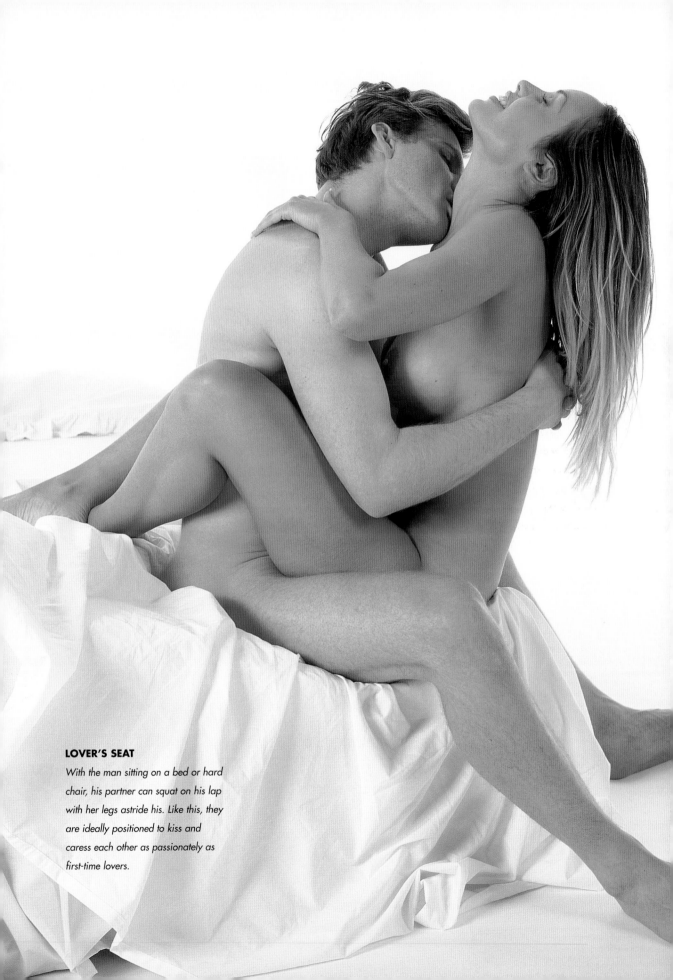

LOVER'S SEAT

With the man sitting on a bed or hard chair, his partner can squat on his lap with her legs astride his. Like this, they are ideally positioned to kiss and caress each other as passionately as first-time lovers.

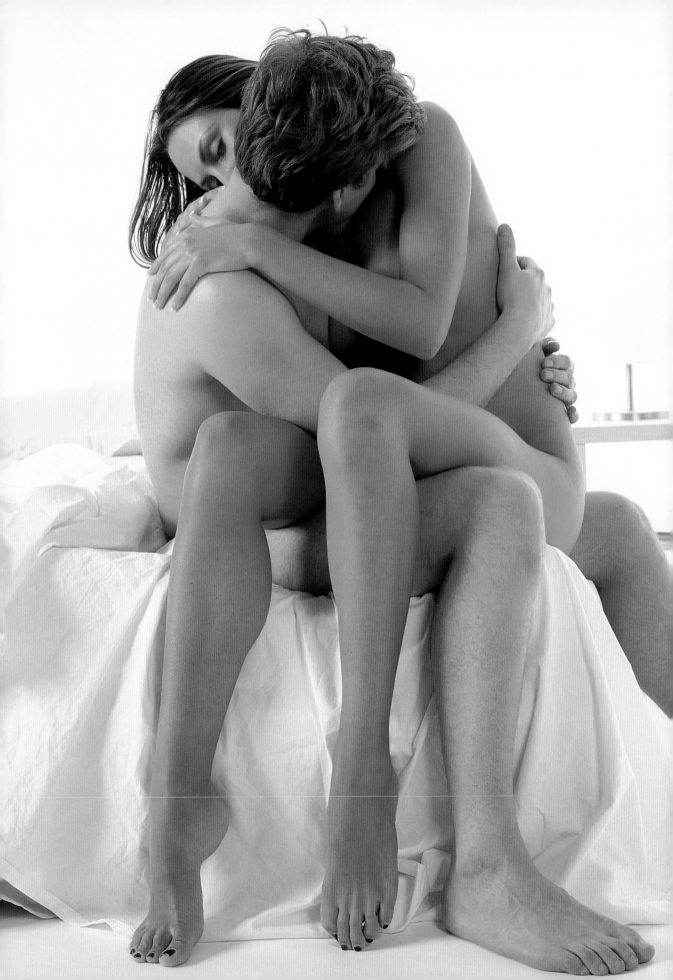

safety first

Always keep safety in mind whenever you are trying out an energetic or adventurous sexual position.

- **Do make sure you are fit enough to cope with some of the positions that require a degree of strength and suppleness. Try some of the 'sexercises', see pages 24–9, before you begin.**

- **Do make sure doors are firmly secured before you lean up against them.**

- **Do push sofas and chairs against a wall so they can't tip back.**

- **Do place cushions and pillows on the floor to protect you – for example, if there is a risk of falling from the edge of a bed.**

- **Don't coerce a partner into trying a position he or she is unhappy about.**

- **Don't adopt a position that causes pain or risks injury.**

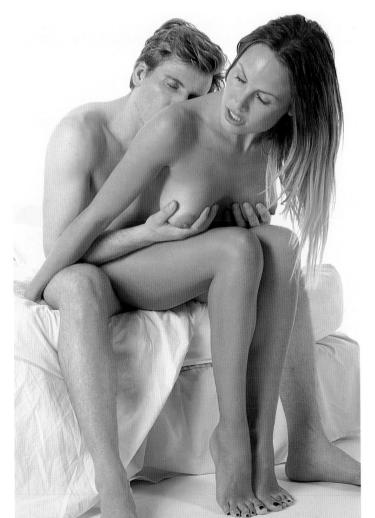

SIDE SADDLE

OPPOSITE: *As a fun variation of chair sex, the woman can sit sideways across her partner's lap, wriggling wildly to enhance the stimulation. In this position, her genital area is easily accessible to manual stimulation. As movement is more restricted, it is ideal for prolonging sex.*

BACK TO FRONT

For a change of direction, the woman can sit facing away from her man, lening forward and holding his upper thighs for support as she rocks her hips, to gain all the advantages of rear-entry sex.

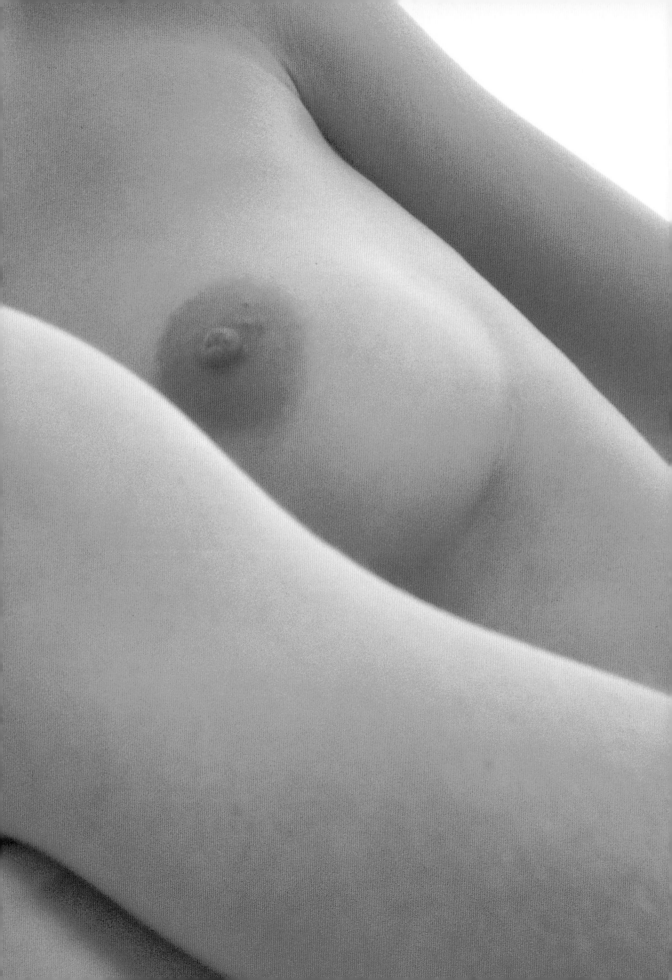

10

DIVINE
SEX

MANY COUPLES SEEK A SPIRITUAL DIMENSION TO SEX, BOTH TO ENHANCE THEIR

RELATIONSHIP AND TO DRAW ON THE INNER LIFE ENERGY THAT IS SAID TO EXIST

INSIDE ALL OF US. ONE WAY IS THROUGH INDIAN MYSTICISM, WHERE THE ACT

OF LOVE IS SEEN AS THE ULTIMATE EXPRESSION OF THE SACRED UNION

BETWEEN MAN AND WOMAN.

tip

Use an artificial lubricant (available from pharmacies) if your vagina tends to become dry or sore, especially during extended lovemaking.

KAMA SUTRA

To many people, Indian lovemaking is synonymous with a book called the Kama Sutra, which means the 'rules of desire'. An Indian sage called Vatsyayana Maharishi, or 'Vatsyayana the Great Seer', wrote this text in the fourth century AD. It describes 64 sexual arts, known as the 'Chatushshashti', and includes eight ways to kiss. Vatsyayana regarded sex as a 'divine union' and a 'celebration of the act of creation'. He advocated explicit sex education for men and women before marriage and believed that intercourse was never sinful, unless done badly!

Many of the practices that Vatsyayana described, such as foreplay, oral sex, and females adopting the woman-on-top position, were regarded as shocking by most Westerners until well into the twentieth century, but are now considered unexceptional. Vatsyayana knew that women were capable of multiple orgasms and stressed the need to ensure that the woman enjoyed sex as much, if not more, than the man – with the aid of an artificial penis, or dildo, if necessary. Many of the positions in the Kama Sutra are designed to prolong sex until the female partner is fully satisfied. By taking a more leisurely approach to lovemaking, both partners can enjoy sex to the full, show their emotional commitment to the relationship and enhance their feelings of intimacy. A sensitive lover learns more about his partner's needs and can ensure that she is fully satisfied before he climaxes.

TANTRA

The spiritual side of lovemaking sees its greatest expression in tantric sex. Tantra, which means 'divine path', emphasizes the more meditative aspect of lovemaking and the prolongation of intercourse. Orgasm is seen as a waste of life energy, which instead should be used to transport the lovers' spiritual consciousness to a far higher plane. Sex represents the fusion of opposites – the male (active) principle with the female (passive) principle – that lies at the heart of nature. By suppressing their selfish desires, and employing special breathing and meditation techniques, a couple can allow their physical, emotional and spiritual energies to merge and achieve a much deeper level of sharing, honesty and understanding.

EXTENDED SEX

Prolonging sex is easier for a woman as she can take four times as long as a man to climax and is capable of multiple orgasms. A couple's main aim, therefore, is to delay the man's orgasm by limiting the level of

TWO HEARTS AS ONE ...

OPPOSITE: *For a more spiritual approach to sex, try meditation. Keep your breathing deep and regular, and free your mind of all distractions. Still breathing deeply, place a hand on your partner's heart. Let your breathing synchronize until you are two hearts beating as one.*

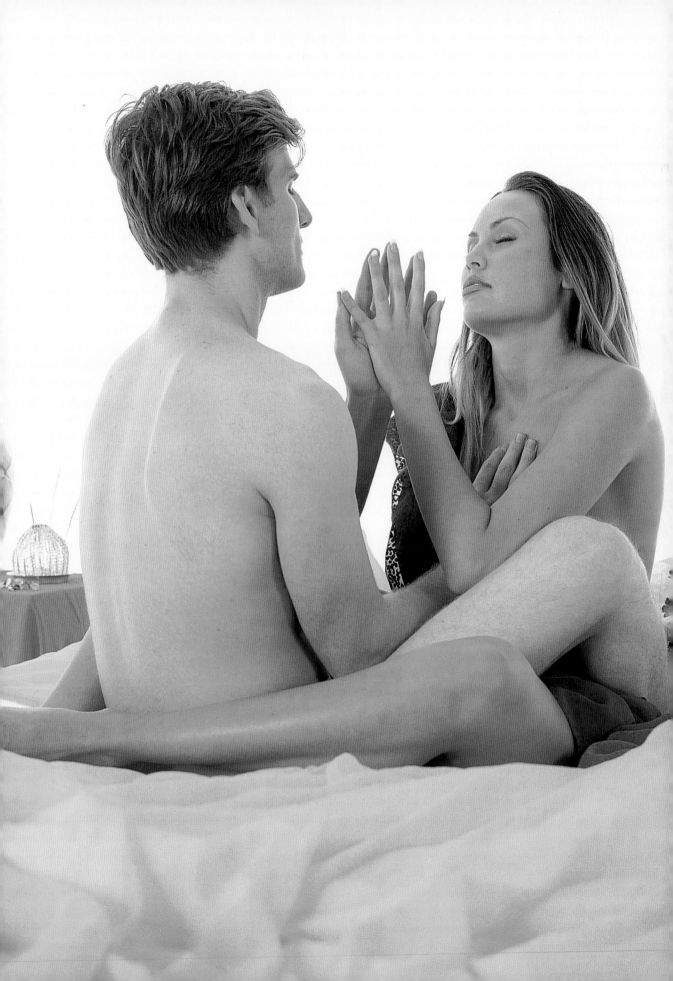

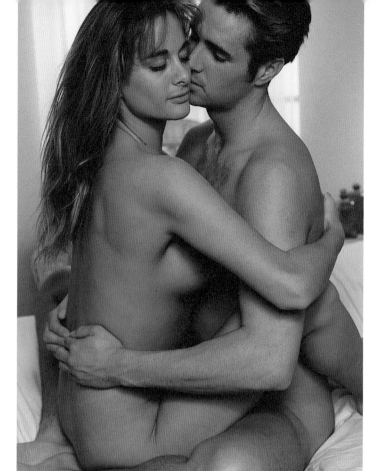

LIFE ENERGY ...

Breathing deeply, lean closer as you join in sexual union. With each in-breath, feel your partner's life energy flowing into you. With each out-breath, feel your life energy flowing into your partner. With practice, you can learn to stay in this position for extended periods of time, showing your reverence for your partner's body with gentle kisses and loving hand caresses.

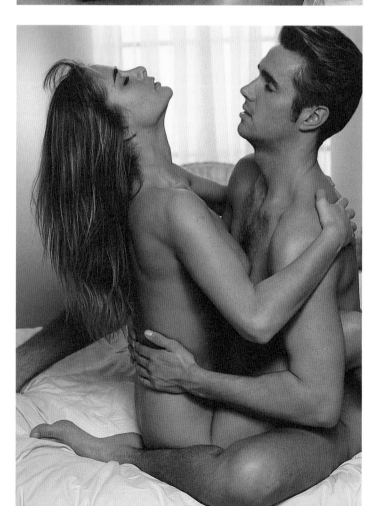

SPIRITUAL CLIMAX

As your sense of oneness develops, together you will experience a physical and spiritual climax in a simultaneous outpouring of sexual ecstasy.

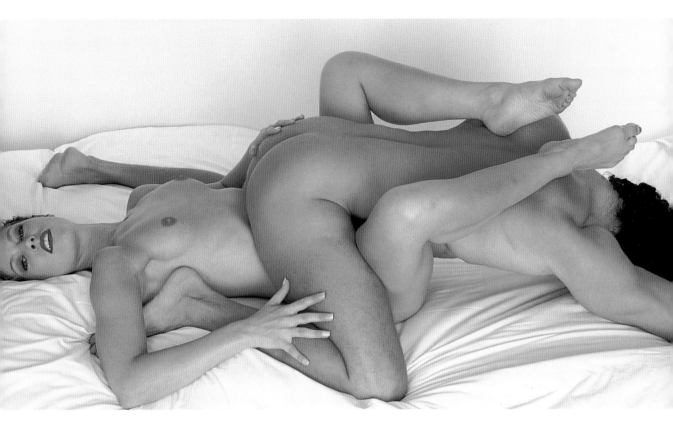

stimulation that he receives. Eastern lovemaking techniques include many ways of achieving this. One method is to keep breathing deeply and to use slow pelvic thrusts. Positions in which a man's movements are greatly restricted can prevent him from accelerating his pelvic movements and so reaching the point of climax too soon. The strongest

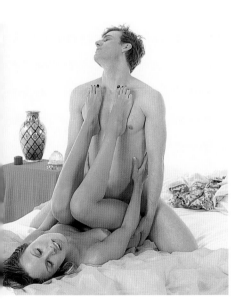

penile stimulation occurs with rapid, shallow thrusting, and so slow, deep penetration helps to delay the man's orgasm. This is because the penis is at its most sensitive toward its tip, and the vagina tightest (and most sensitive) near its entrance. The woman needs to be aware of her partner's state of arousal so that she can slow down the pace and, if necessary, allow his penis to penetrate her more deeply. Positions such as the woman on top, in which she is in complete control, can help here.

A NEW SLANT

A very difficult position, but one that allows a unique form of stimulation. The man penetrates his partner in reverse and achieves novel sensations by thrusting back.

KAMA CLASSIC

In this classic pose from the Kama Sutra, the woman's knees are raised, her legs are together and her feet resting on the man's chest. The man is able to penetrate her slowly and deeply in this position.

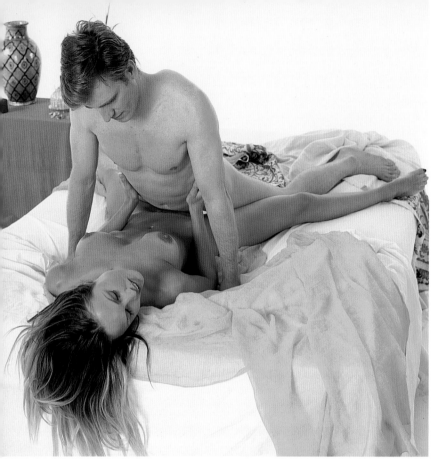

OPEN WIDE

Another pose from the Kama Sutra. Here, the woman lies on her back with her legs straight and very wide apart. The man's legs are also very wide apart, allowing only slow, rhythmic thrusting movements of his pelvis.

SLOW MOTION

BELOW: *The woman sits astride the man in the 'Reverse St George' position (see page 68) and then leans back so that she is resting on his chest. It is difficult for him to move his pelvis, but he can caress his partner's breasts and clitoris.*

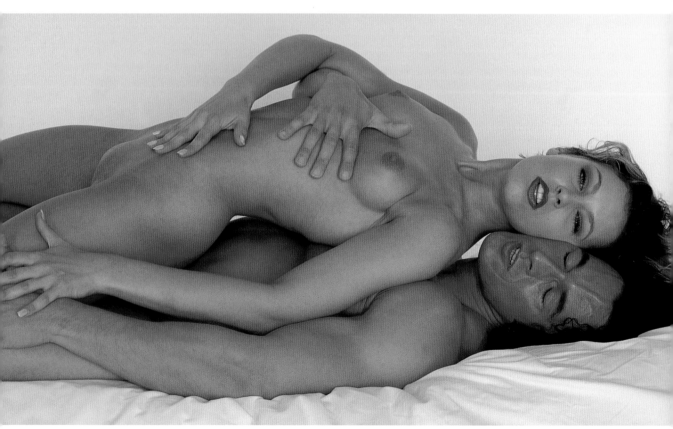

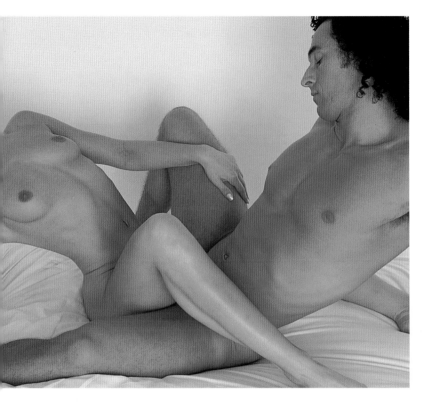

X-POSE

In this position, each partner lies with one leg over and one under their partner's leg. Movement is greatly restricted, so this position is ideal for slow, extended lovemaking. By coordinating their movements, the man can maintain his erection for longer to give his partner time to climax. This pose also ensures greater stimulation of the sensitive perineum.

FLAT OUT

Here, the woman lies on top of the man, resting her feet on his. This position ensures maximum skin-to-skin contact, but minimal movement so that the friction of their genitals remains at the lowest level of stimulation.

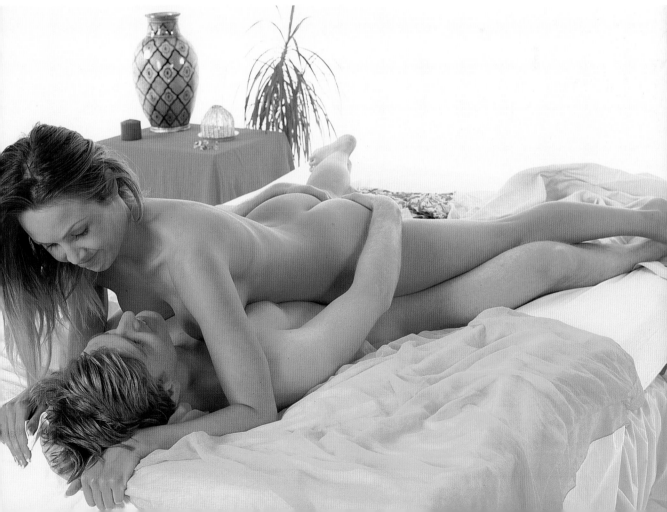

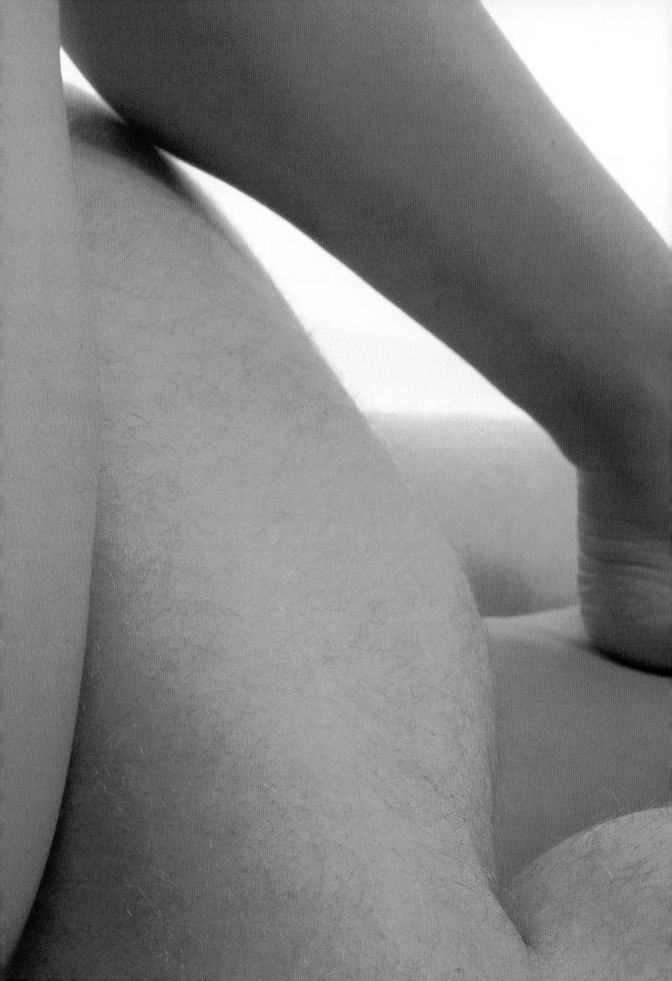

11

DREAM LOVERS

THE POWER OF THE MIND AND, ESPECIALLY, THE IMAGINATION, IS A VITAL

PART OF SEX. EROTIC THOUGHTS NOT ONLY TRIGGER AROUSAL, THEY ALSO ENSURE

THAT SEXUAL FEELINGS ARE MAINTAINED AND STEADILY BUILD TO A CLIMAX.

BY MAKING THE MOST OF THE 'SEXUAL MIND', COUPLES CAN TAKE THEIR

LOVEMAKING TO NEW HEIGHTS.

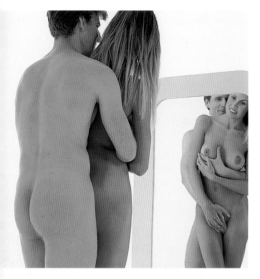

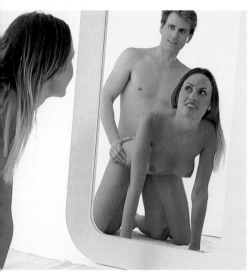

MIRROR MAGIC

Placing a mirror near your bed – or over it – can give a unique view of your partner's body and allows you to see the pleasure on your own face as you enjoy your lover's embrace. Suddenly you are both 'voyeurs' – eager spectators as well as enthusiastic participants in your own lovemaking – and loving every second of it.

THE SEXUAL MIND

The most important sexual organ of all is the brain, and the many complex and interconnected areas of the brain that are involved in sexual arousal can be thought of as the 'sexual mind'. There are special nerve pathways that link the sexual mind with the genitals and other erogenous zones through a feedback system. The signals that travel up or down these pathways can either increase your sexual excitement (positive feedback), or decrease it (negative feedback). For example, memories, erotic images and sounds, the sight, voice and feel of a lover can all reinforce arousal. Tension, anxiety, stress, guilt, fear, self-doubt and poor self-image, however, can inhibit sexual feelings. If couples do not use the power of the mind to the full, sex can become a dull, mechanical process that quickly loses its magic.

Prepare for love

Before you start to make love, ensure you are both mentally prepared for it by taking enough time to relax, shutting out all other distractions and getting into a more sexy mood. An element of fun and fantasy is important to many people, helping them to get aroused and increasing their enjoyment of sex. Most people have a few fantasies that they want to keep to themselves, and this is perfectly understandable. But it can be fun to share your secret fantasy with your partner and to construct erotic visions that you can talk about together, or even create a sexual scenario that you can act out with your lover. Only the breadth of your imagination limits your choice of play.

Arousing apparel

Clothing is a powerful sexual trigger for many men and women. Tight trousers or shorts, see-through blouses, boxer shorts, stockings and suspenders, can all act to 'release' sexual feelings in many people. Sometimes it is the feel of a particular material, such as rubber, leather, lace or silk, that has the desired effect. The origins of these sexual triggers often lie in childhood or adolescence and usually remain buried in the depths of the subconscious. They are nothing to be ashamed of, so don't feel inhibited about telling your partner that you're turned on by a particular item or style of clothing. And encourage your partner to discuss his or her tastes with you. Conflicts in relationships are more often due to poor communication than openness.

Erotica

Many couples enjoy viewing erotic material such as magazines, books or films together. These images are, in effect, sexual fantasies that are being acted out by others for your benefit. Whether a particular scenario works for you depends on your personal likes and dislikes. It may be sufficient for a man just to view an explicit sexual image or scene, whereas a woman often needs to have a sexy, plausible story line and attractive, likeable characters to give the erotic imagery a human dimension. Talking about your own sexual preferences and finding out what really excites your lover can offer a truly fascinating insight into a partner's sexual psyche.

Some couples like to video their own erotic scenes to view at a later time. A simpler way to see yourself performing is to make love in front of a large mirror. You may find that sex becomes a more exciting experience as, for the first time, you see yourself getting aroused and can watch the movements of your body in your lover's embrace.

ADULT GAMES

Be the femme fatale you've always wanted to be. Now that you've removed your own clothes, it's time to start undressing your partner. To prolong the fun, try undoing his trousers with your teeth.

tip

Women who prepare themselves mentally for a romantic liaison by fantasizing about the event beforehand find they are more easily aroused and more likely to be sexually satisfied than those who do not.

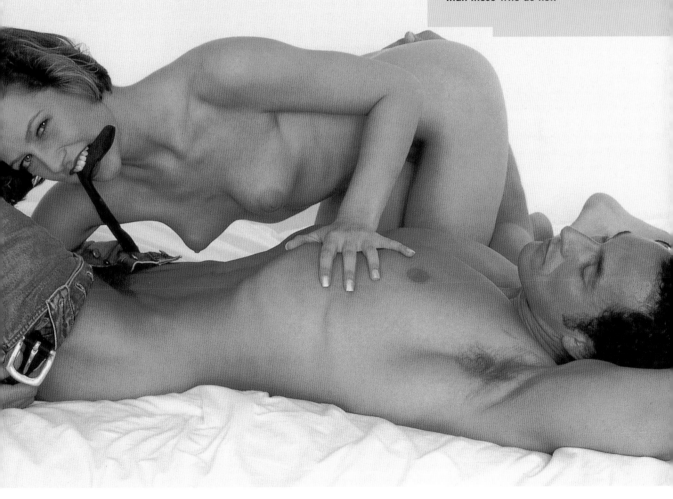

SEXY UNDERWEAR

The combination of a sexy bra, knickers, stockings and suspenders can be a powerful turn-on for your partner and a sexually liberating experience for you, especially if you don't usually wear these items.

EROTIC IMAGERY

Looking at an erotic magazine together offers an opportunity to discuss your sexual likes and dislikes. It can be a real eye-opener for men to discover what women really like to see. Be prepared to be surprised.

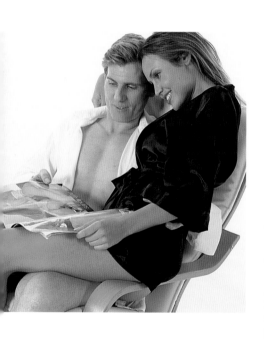

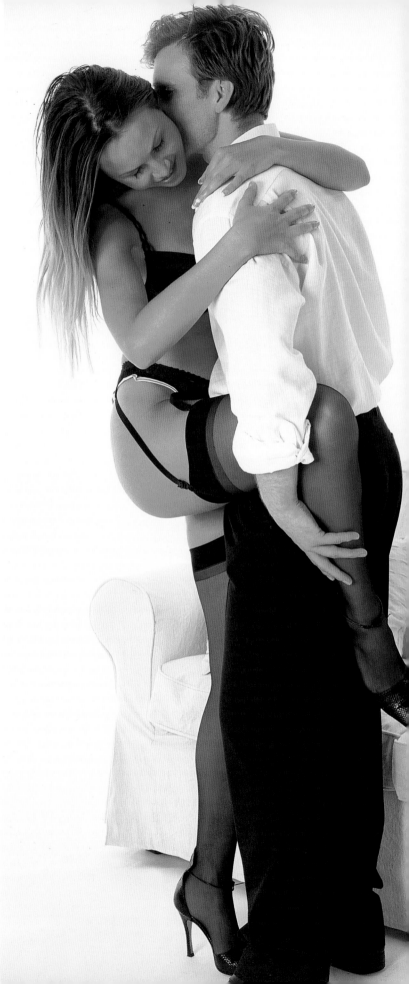

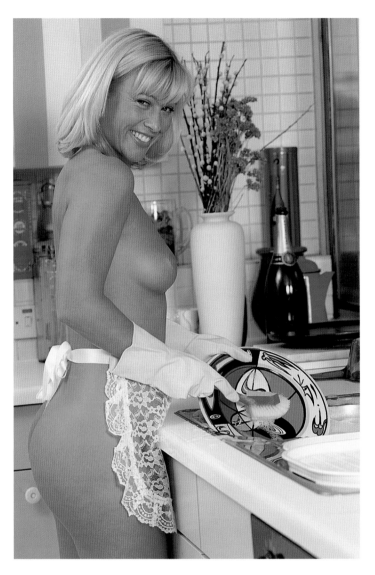

FUN CHORES
Even the most mundane chores are great fun when you introduce a sexy element to the task.

MASKS
A 'masquerade' mask adds an air of mystery to lovemaking. Through the power of your imagination, your partner is transformed into whoever you want him, or her, to be.

SECRET STRIPPER

One way a woman can reveal her sexy side, and have fun as well, is to perform a striptease for her partner. She'll enjoy the expression on his face as, when he's least expecting it, she starts to gyrate in front of him, peeling off layers of clothing to a background of raunchy music. The man need not be left out, either. Another time it can be his turn to perform, as a male stripper, disrobing before a wide-eyed and enthusiastic 'hen-night audience' of one. Striptease is just one form of role-play that couples can use to bring sexual fantasies to life. Another is to dress up as a movie idol, or a character in a TV show or sexy advert, and use their imagination to become the screen god and goddess they've always wanted to be.

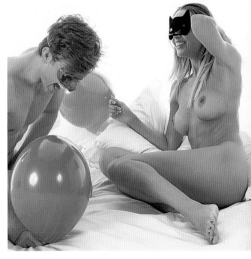

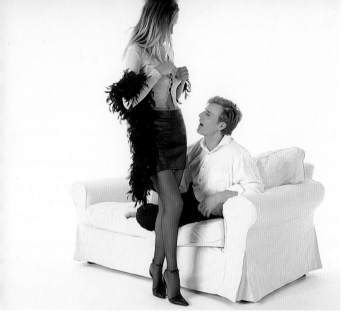

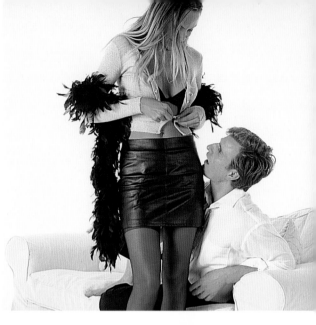

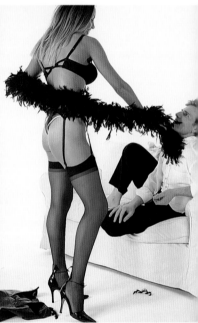

STRIPTEASE TEMPTRESS

As a stripper, you can let your sexy side emerge.
Dress up in your most provocative clothes, put on
some sexy music and move your body to the beat.
This is a chance to really show off your raunchy nature
as, swaying provocatively, you slowly and sexily remove
each delicate piece of clothing, one by one. Remember,
this is a tease, as well as a strip, so take your time.
You are a performer, even though you are only
appearing in front of an audience of one. Encourage
your partner, but don't let him get too involved – just
yet. By the time the last item of clothing is removed,
the eager spectator will be keen to move on to the
next stage of the evening's performance, where he
can take a more active part!

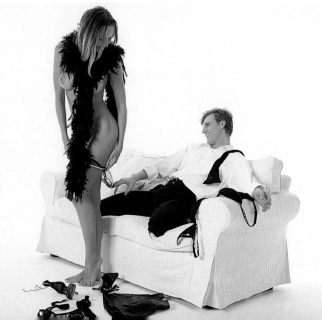

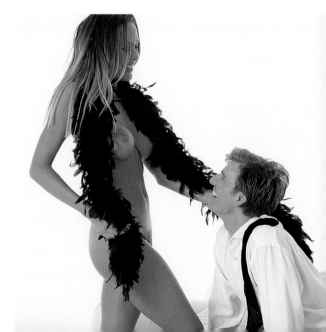

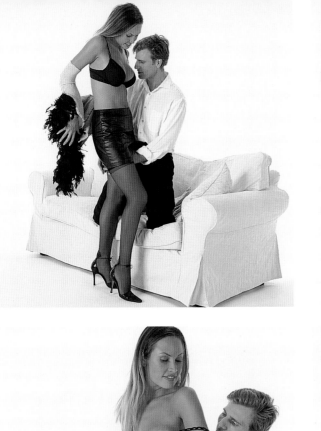
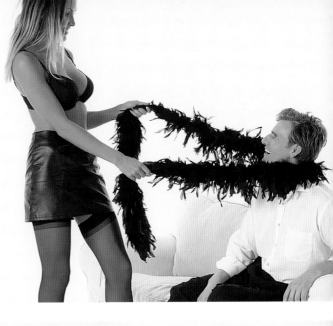
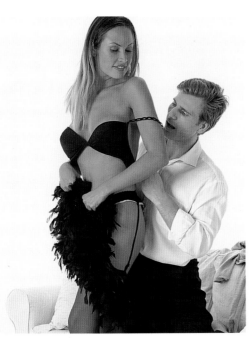
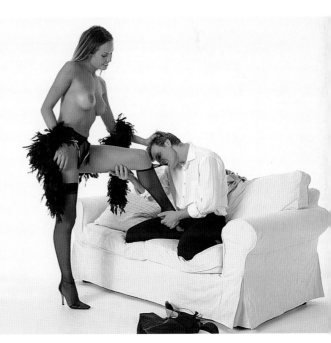
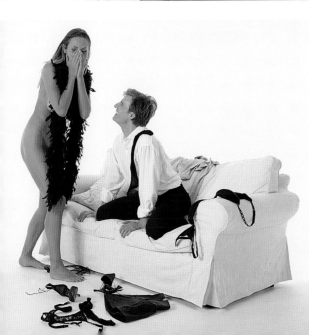
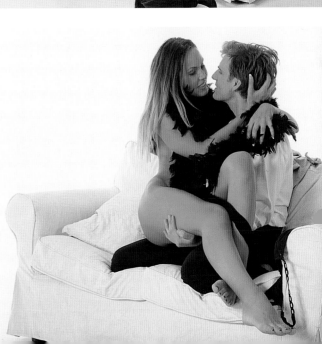

MOTOR MAN

A car mechanic – with overall charm! If your partner normally only sees you in chinos, or a suit and tie, revealing this new side of yourself will be a nice surprise for her.

GIRL BUILDER

Whatever your personal fantasy, it's fun to act it out through role-play. You don't necessarily need props, such as a hard hat, but they may help you get into character.

EASY RIDER

If a biker in a leather jacket seems like the answer to your dreams, suggest it to your partner – and let him speed you to paradise.

FRENCH MAID

OPPOSITE: There's something about a French maid's dress that brings out the Parisian in every man. (And housework is not usually at the top of the agenda.)

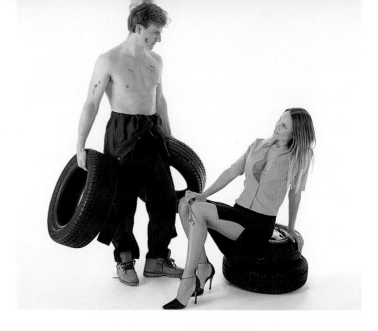

top female fantasies

These are the most popular female fantasies, as reported in surveys:

- Making love with a current partner.
- Making love with former lovers.
- Making love with a movie star or other famous man.
- Making love in romantic, exotic or unusual locations.
- Receiving oral sex.
- Being an irresistible sexual temptress.
- Mild sado-masochistic sex (bondage, spanking).

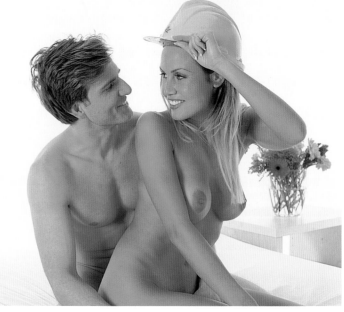

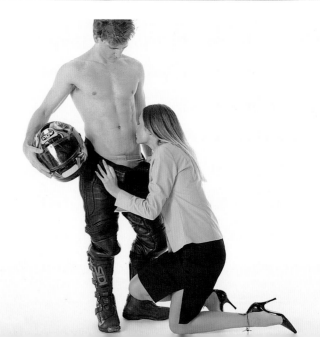

top male fantasies

These are the most popular male fantasies, as reported in surveys:

- Making love with a current partner.
- Making love with former lovers.
- Group sex.
- Partner swapping.
- Watching others have sex.
- Being sexually dominant.
- Mild sado-masochistic sex (bondage, spanking).

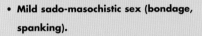

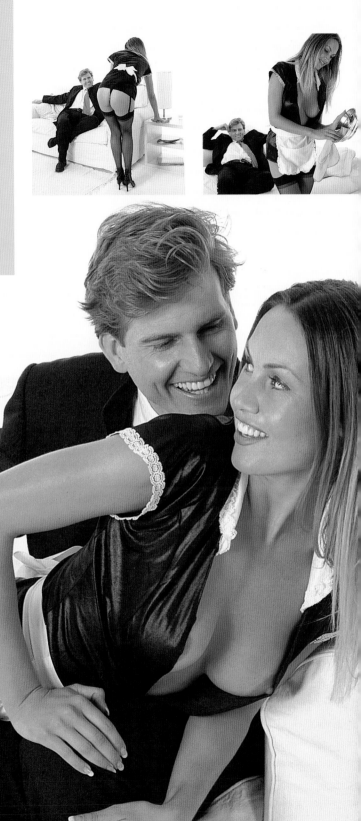

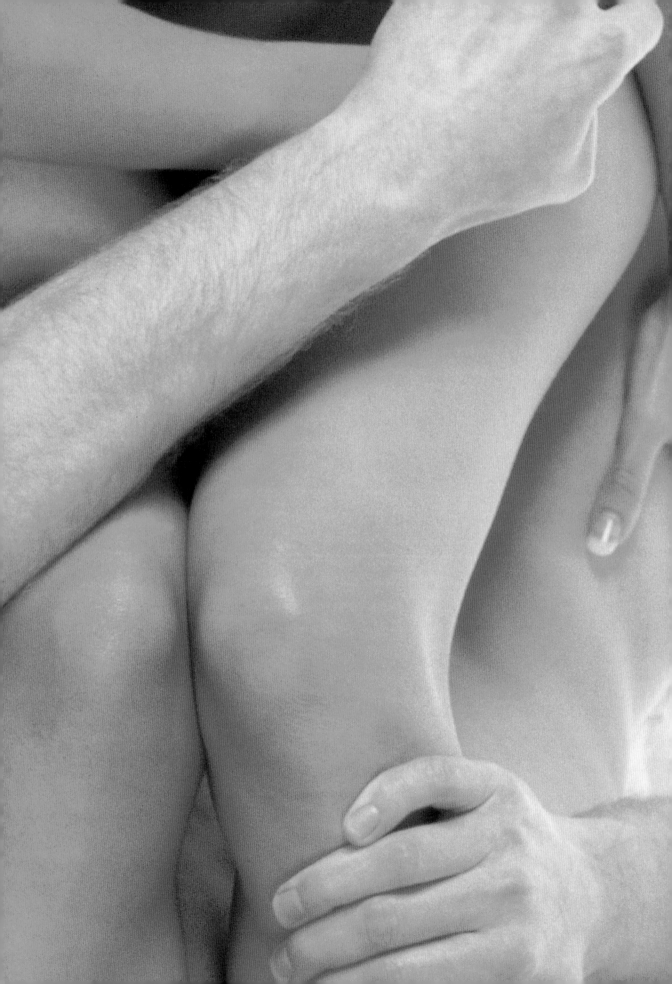

12

FUN AND GAMES

LOVE GAMES LET COUPLES ENJOY FUN, PLAYFUL LOVEMAKING AND HELP THEM

TO BREAK FREE FROM THE PRESSURES AND TENSIONS OF 'SERIOUS SEX'. THROUGH

PLAY, MEN AND WOMEN BECOME MORE INVENTIVE, SEEKING EXCITING

NEW SENSATIONS TO BEGUILE THEIR SENSES AND ENJOYING A HEDONISTIC

ORGY OF SENSUAL DELIGHTS.

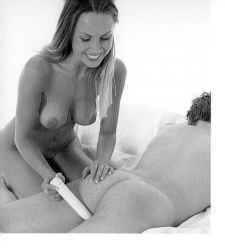

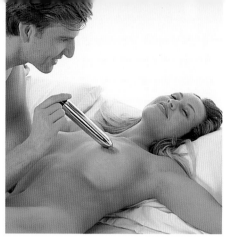

GOOD VIBRATIONS

ABOVE LEFT: *As a fun addition to foreplay, apply a vibrator to your partner's perineum to increase his enjoyment of sex.*

WONDER WEAPON

ABOVE RIGHT: *You'll find that a vibrator is a powerful device to hold in your hands when you place it against your partner's naked skin and then gently rub it over the most sexually sensitive parts of her body.*

SOLO STYLE

OPPOSITE: *When you are on your own and feeling aroused, you can discover more about your sexual nature by applying a vibrator to your pubic area, while using your free hand to stimulate other parts of your body.*

sexual hygiene

A vibrator or other device that has been inserted in the anus should always be washed with soap and water before it is placed in or near the vagina. Or cover the device with a condom, which you dispose of.

SEX TOYS

When people think of love games, often the first things that pop into their mind are sex toys. There is now such an amazing abundance of devices available that a visit to a sex shop is like stepping into an Aladdin's cave of rampant sexuality. The oldest sex toy of all is probably the dildo, or artificial penis, which is referred to in the Kama Sutra. Dildos can look highly realistic, but they have exaggerated ribbing for extra stimulation.

The most popular sex toy of all is the vibrator, a battery-operated device, available in a whole range of sizes, that generates powerfully arousing sensations when applied to the body. Many women say that a vibrator offers a reliable way to achieve an orgasm, especially when used to stimulate the clitoris, labia or perineum, or when inserted into the vagina. Men, too, enjoy the sensations a vibrator produces when placed against the penis, scrotum, perineum or anus.

Vibrators are available in a range of sizes and shapes. Most are roughly penis-shaped, but some are egg-shaped and can be placed inside the vagina. Love balls are covered metal balls, usually non-powered, that are inserted into the vagina and left in place. They move against each other, stimulating pleasurable sensations for the woman. A clitoral stimulator is an aid to penetrative sex. It is a ring-shaped device that fits around the penis and has a small projection that rubs against the clitoris with every thrusting movement.

Homemade fun

You needn't go to a sex shop for sex aids. Take a look around your own home, where you'll find plenty of objects that, with a little imagination, provide unusual and arousing stimulation. The most powerful sensations can be created through a contrast of temperatures. It can be highly arousing for a man to, say, rub an ice cube over his partner's nipple, or for a woman to suck an ice cream and then take her lover's penis in her mouth. A stiff feather drawn lightly over the inner thigh or vulva can make a partner wriggle with delight, and a hair dryer – set on cold – is a fun addition to playful sex. A man can use it on its lowest setting to blow gently over his partner's skin while she is still damp from a shower. Alternatively, he can simply moisten her skin with his mouth and tongue, and blow across it with pursed lips.

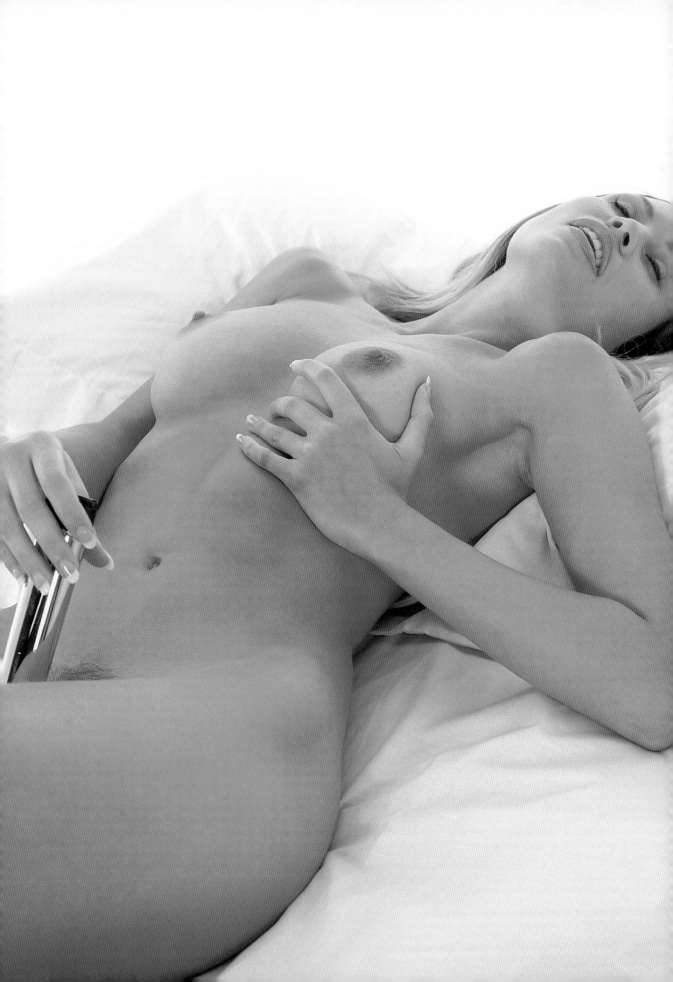

sex game – for his eyes only

Cover your partner's eyes with a blindfold. Part her legs and then slowly – and teasingly – run your hands over her breasts and abdomen, down to her pubic mound, and along the insides of her thighs (avoiding her vulva). Carry on stroking her body, but still avoiding her genitals, as she slowly gets aroused. Pause for a few seconds to increase her sense of expectation. Then, without touching any other part of her body, brush your finger lightly along her vulva. If you've timed it right, she'll gasp and an intensely pleasurable feeling, like a mild electric shock, will pass through her body.

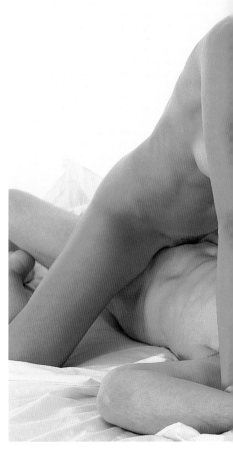

TOTAL SUBMISSION

Straddling your partner, with his hands held firmly above his head, you dictate the pace and style of lovemaking as he lies helplessly, and happily, below you.

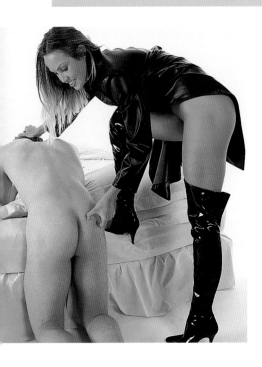

POWER GAMES

Partners who usually have equal roles during intercourse can get a special thrill out of playing power or fun fetish games, such as domination, bondage and spanking. Some people find that being completely submissive to a partner can free their minds of any guilt associations with sex that may have arisen in childhood so they can simply abandon themselves to their lover. Others like the thrill of exercising control over their partner. Then they, in turn, can allow their partner to take charge of their sexual arousal.

OBEY YOUR MISTRESS

Many men are surprised at the enjoyment they gain by submitting themselves to their partner's will, giving her a free hand – literally – to find new and inventive ways to stimulate his body.

It is important to remember that this is just a game conducted for pure pleasure, though, in which both partners are regarded as willing accomplices. One partner submits to the other's domination only because he or she consents. As you're just play-acting, for games of bondage, it's only necessary to tie or loop ribbons or pieces of silk loosely around wrists and ankles. Then, if either partner wishes to end the game at any stage, they can release themselves easily.

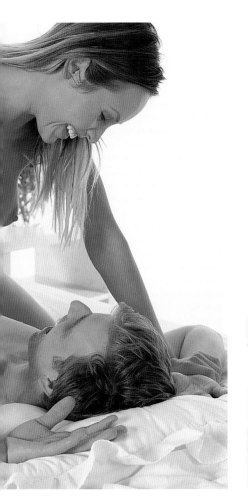

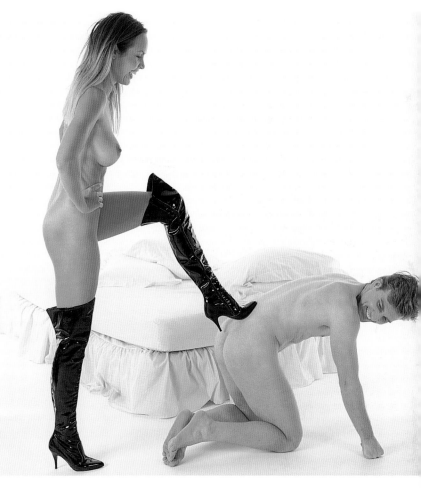

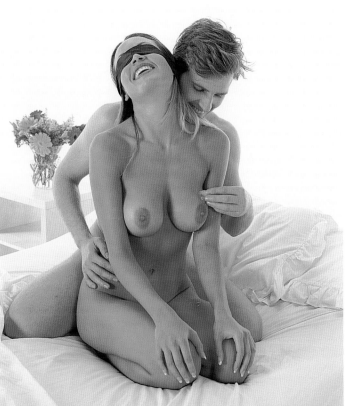

THE DOMINATRIX

A woman may find she gets a sexual thrill through donning knee-length leather boots and other items of the Dominatrix and 'forcing' her naked partner to do her every bidding.

ICE IS NICE

The cold sensation of an ice cube rubbed gently over your partner's nipple can be an amazingly erotic sensation for her – and you can warm it up again afterwards with your mouth.

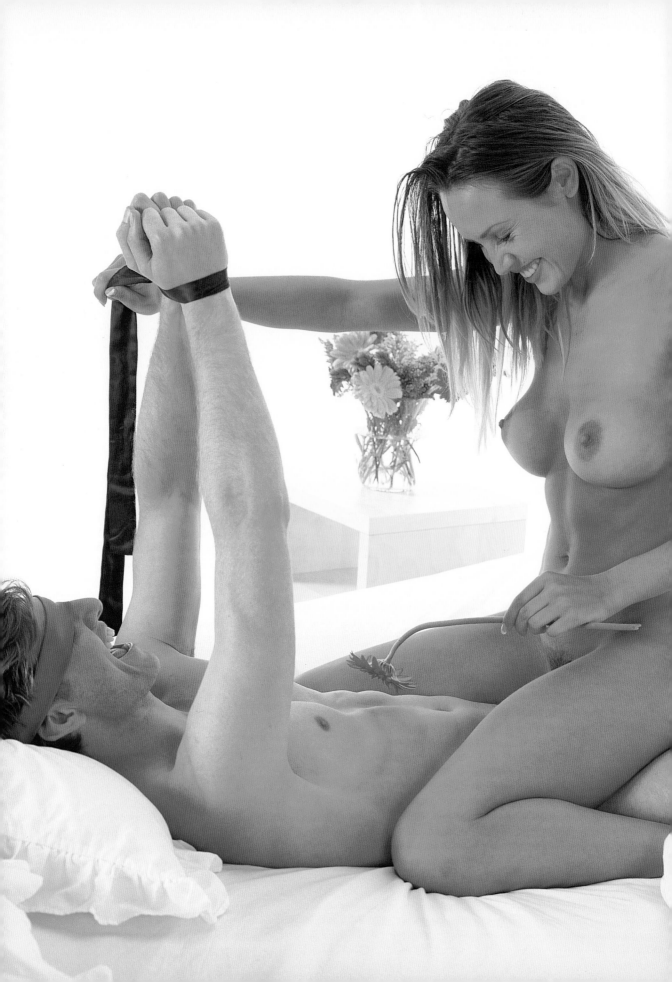

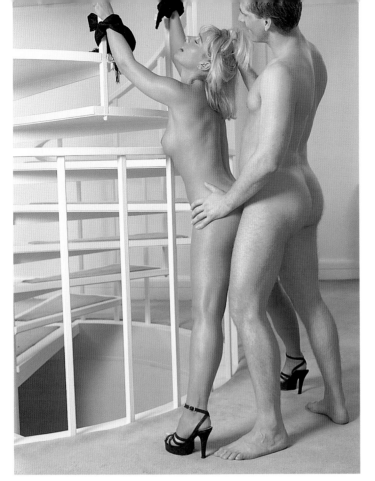

BONDAGE BOYS AND BABES

LEFT AND OPPOSITE: *You're in charge – so make the most of it. Tease and arouse your lover and then, as they near orgasm, suddenly slow down and make them beg for more.*

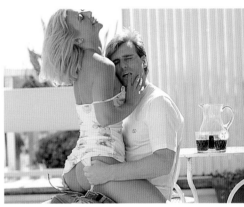

AL FRESCO SEX

For the zest of dangerous sex, make love in the garden. This could remain a fantasy that you share only with your lover – unless you have the courage to do it for real!

STAIRWAY TO HEAVEN

Make love in different places – in the hall, on the kitchen floor or on the stairs, wherever you can think of that will add a sparkle to your love life.

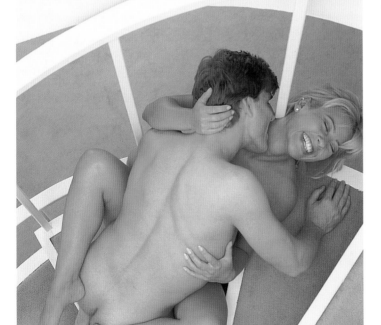

safety tips

For safety's sake:

• Never use a mains-powered hair dryer in the bathroom as there is a serious risk of electrocution.

• Never blow air into the ears, mouth, nose or vagina – with the mouth, or a mechanical device, such as a hair dryer or air pump – as there is a danger of forcing an air bubble into the bloodstream, with potentially fatal consequences.

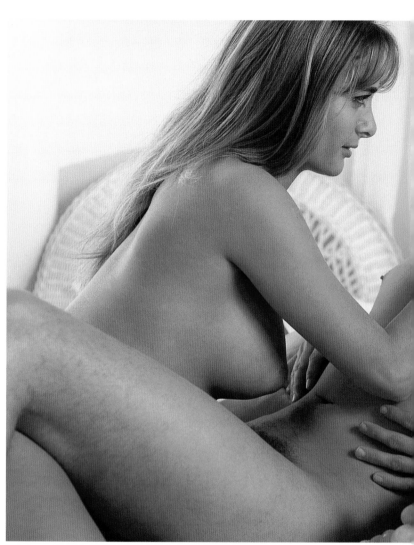

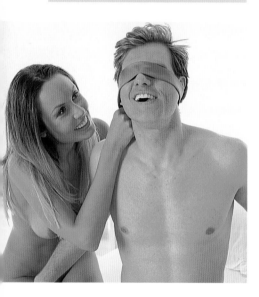

HIDDEN PLEASURES

With your partner blindfolded, experiment with new sensations. This will help to strengthen the bond of trust between you.

CREAMY DELIGHT

Enjoy a fantasy feast, using your partner as a plate. Squirt cream from a spray can over her body, then take your time to lick it off with the tip of your tongue.

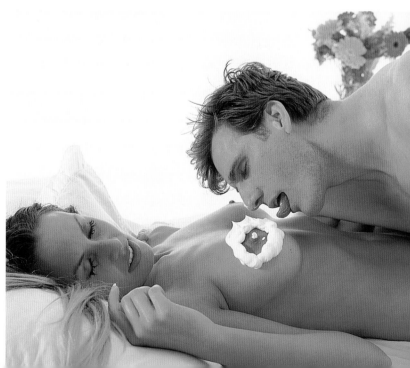

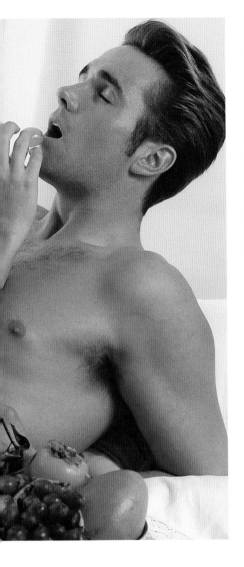

GET FRUITY

Have your very own Roman orgy and tickle your partner's tastebuds by feeding him the most mouthwatering morsels you can find.

JUST A QUICKIE

Submit to the electrifying power of raw, quickie sex. If you're so aroused that there is just no time to reach the bedroom, make love whenever and wherever the mood takes you.

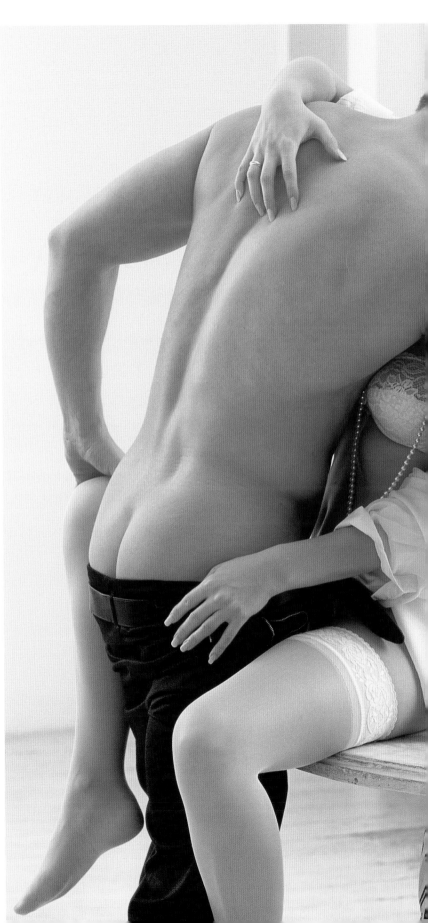

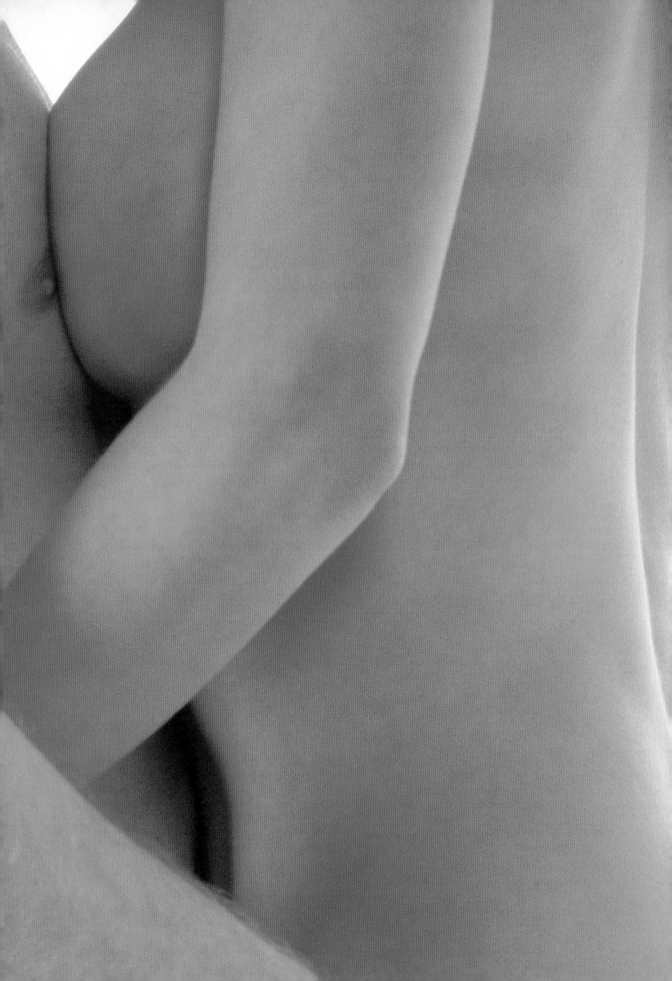

OVERCOMING PROBLEMS

SEXUAL PROBLEMS CAN DEVELOP AT ANY TIME OF LIFE, AND FOR ALL SORTS OF REASONS.

WITH PATIENCE AND UNDERSTANDING, COUPLES CAN RESOLVE PROBLEMS WHEN THEY

FIRST ARISE, OR LEARN HOW TO ADAPT TO CHANGING CIRCUMSTANCES WHILE

MAINTAINING A LOVING, SHARING AND SATISFYING SEXUAL RELATIONSHIP.

A PROBLEM SHARED

Sexual problems should never be suffered in silence. In many cases, difficulties can be resolved simply by talking them through together. Family doctors are trained to deal with sexual and relationship issues, or they can refer couples on to an expert. The doctor may diagnose an underlying cause, such as diabetes, that requires medical attention, and/or suggest sex therapy or relationship counselling. Always seek medical advice if a sexual problem is affecting your relationship.

FEMALE SEXUAL PROBLEMS

A common sexual problem in women is pain during intercourse (sexual pain disorder or dispareunia). Sex should never be painful, but in a young female, especially, a lack of knowledge about her sexual nature, combined with inhibition and fear of being hurt or of getting pregnant, can cause her to become tense during sex, resulting in pain. In more severe cases, a woman may suffer painful spasms of the vaginal walls.

Other causes of sexual pain, such as vaginal dryness, and problems like reduced libido (sexual desire disorder), inability to become sexually excited (sexual arousal disorder) or inability to climax (orgasmic disorder), may be due to poor sexual technique, psychological issues, physical disorders or relationship difficulties. Sex during pregnancy raises its own special concerns, too (see opposite).

Painful intercourse

In many cases, pain during intercourse is due to vaginal dryness, and this may be a sign that a woman is not sufficiently aroused to allow penetrative sex. This can be avoided if her partner spends more time on foreplay and other techniques that ensure she is fully sexually stimulated.

Vaginal dryness can also occur following childbirth, or in later life when the vaginal tissues become thinner and produce less lubrication. If the problem persists, the woman should see a doctor. A short-term remedy may be to use an artificial lubricant, such as a water-based gel, available from pharmacies. (Saliva may work as a temporary measure.) In some cases, pain is due to a physical disorder, such as bartholinitis (inflammation of the Bartholin's glands, on either side of the vaginal entrance), requiring medical treatment.

Vaginismus

In this condition, a woman is prevented from having intercourse because the muscular walls of her vagina go into spasm whenever a penis, or even a finger, is pushed inside her. It may be due to a physical disorder, or a traumatic event in the past that has caused her to link sex (or other contact with her genitals) with pain. Other psychological or emotional factors can play a part, too. For example, a woman may feel guilty or anxious about sex, perhaps because of upbringing or religious or cultural taboos. It is important to consult a doctor to discover the underlying cause of vaginismus.

Self-help for vaginismus

Here, self-help techniques may be beneficial. For example, a woman can use a mirror to explore her genitals with her fingers and learn how to relax her genital muscles. Once she is used to the touch of her own fingers, she can ask her partner to stroke her with his fingers, without progressing to sex, until she no longer tenses up at his touch.

A sex therapist can provide vaginal trainers (plastic rods ranging from finger-size to larger devices) that are used to practise widening the vagina. At first, the woman tries to relax enough to use the smallest device. When she has mastered this, she moves on to the next size. Once she feels relaxed enough for penetrative sex, she should try the woman-on-top position (see pages 66 and 68) so she can control the pace and depth of penetration.

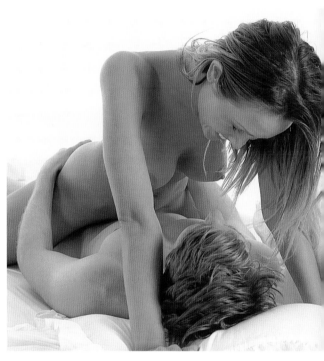

SEXUAL RELEASE

Many women find it difficult to really let go during sex. Try to clear your mind of nagging worries and feelings of guilt and just go with the flow ...

Positions for pregnancy

Many pregnant women experience an increase in sexual desire, due to the higher levels of circulating hormones in the body, but worry that sex is unsafe during pregnancy. In fact, studies show that careful intercourse does no harm at all to mother or baby, even after the 29th week of pregnancy, and may increase the likelihood that a pregnancy continues to term. But deep penetration and the man-on-top position are best avoided in late pregnancy. The safest positions are side-by-side, spoons and woman on top (see pages 66–71) that put no pressure on the woman's abdomen. If she has a history of miscarriage, a doctor may advise against penetrative sex, but mutual masturbation and oral sex are usually regarded as safe at any stage.

Orgasmic disorders

To climax, a woman must feel comfortable with her surroundings, happy with her partner, good about herself and relaxed about her sexual responses. Only then can she really let herself go. If she feels at all tense, self-conscious or inhibited in any way, she may not be able to have an orgasm. This is why it's important that her partner creates the right mood for sex, knows how to arouse her and devotes enough time to foreplay before attempting intercourse.

A woman may find it difficult to achieve an orgasm through penetrative sex alone, but may find she can do so successfully through manual stimulation. This may be because of psychological or relationship issues, which prevent her from enjoying penetrative sex, or because the penis does not stimulate her enough. In this case, she and her partner should experiment by trying out different positions such as side-by-side, woman on top and spoons (see pages 66–71), that allow the woman or the man to stimulate her clitoris by hand.

Bridge technique
Another approach to the problem is to use the Bridge Technique, which is designed to act as a bridge between manual and penile stimulation, hence the name. The man stimulates his partner's clitoris, vagina and other erogenous areas by using his hands, or a vibrator, for example, until she's close to orgasm. He then enters her and brings her to orgasm with penile thrusting and, if necessary, additional stimulation.

AROUSAL ...

BELOW LEFT: *The Bridge Technique can be effective when a woman has difficulty in achieving orgasm through penetration alone. Her partner arouses her through foreplay and continues to stimulate her manually or with a vibrator.*

... AND CLIMAX

Once the woman is close to orgasm, the man enters her and brings her to orgasm with the thrusting action of his penis.

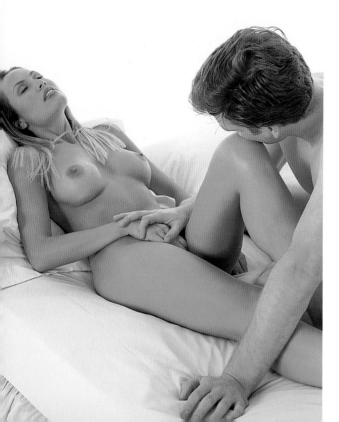
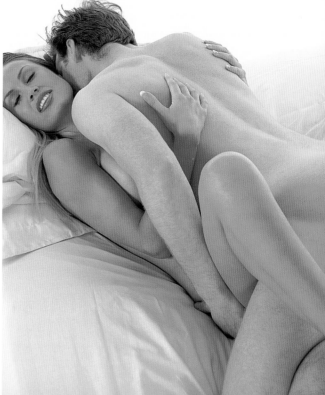

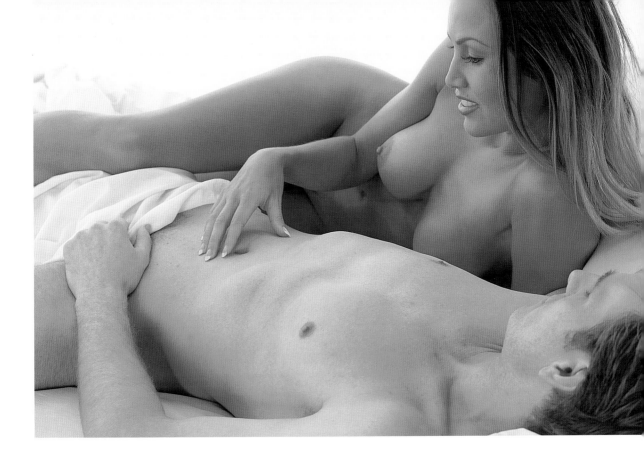

MALE SEXUAL PROBLEMS

Inexperience, tension or over-excitement may cause a man to climax too soon (premature ejaculation) before his partner is sexually satisfied. At various times in his life, stress, anxiety or illness can make it difficult for him to achieve or sustain an erection (impotence or erectile dysfunction), or ejaculate normally (inhibited/retrograde ejaculation).

Factors may combine to create a vicious downward spiral. For example, stress can cause temporary impotence, which may trigger the fear that the problem will recur, thus making the situation worse. Soon, the problem may become chronic, leading to relationship difficulties and further stress.

Ejaculation problems

Premature ejaculation is a common sexual problem. With practice, most men will learn how to delay their orgasm. A man may find that having ejaculated once, he can then prolong his lovemaking more easily during subsequent intercourse. Using a condom can help here, as it reduces the sensitivity of the penis, and there are other techniques he can use (see Chapters 2 and 10). If the problem persists, the couple should seek medical advice to rule out a physical or psychological cause. Sexual therapy or counselling is beneficial in some cases.

SENSATE FOCUS ...

This technique can be helpful in resolving male or female problems. For sensate focus to be effective, the couple need to find times when they can relax and shut out all other distractions. There should be no pressure to perform or achieve a goal. During the early stages, they take turns to touch each other, keeping to non-sexual areas of the body.

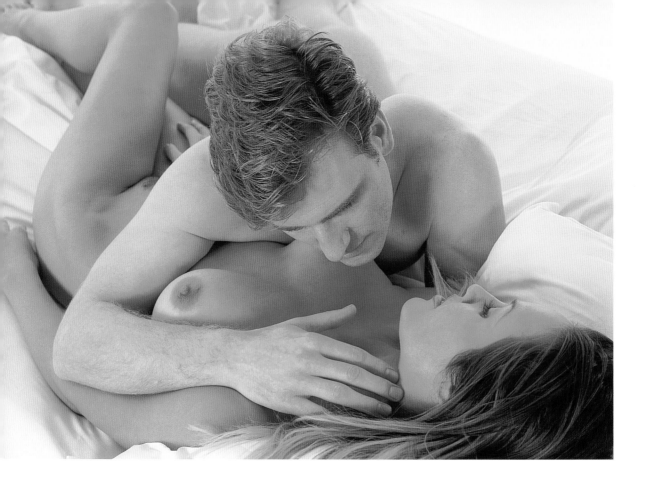

Squeeze technique

Another remedy is the Squeeze Technique. This works best when a woman takes control, straddling her partner in the woman-on-top position (see page 68), for example, and determines the pace and speed of penetration. The man lets the woman know when he's close to ejaculating and his partner grips the top of his penis, with a finger or thumb against the frenulum, and squeezes for four seconds. This action makes the erection subside slightly and delays ejaculation. It is repeated every time he's close to ejaculating, to a maximum of three times. Then he ejaculates as normal. If the technique is used whenever the couple have sex, the man soon learns to delay ejaculation without manual help. The Squeeze can also be applied to the base of the penis.

Other male sexual problems can include inhibited ejaculation, when ejaculation is delayed or fails to occur, and retrograde ejaculation, when semen spurts backwards into the bladder. Inhibited ejaculation may be due to a psychological problem, like anxiety, or a physical problem, such as diabetes, or a side effect of medication. A doctor will advise. Retrograde ejaculation is usually due to neurological disease or pelvic surgery. There is no treatment for this problem, but having a full bladder during intercourse can help.

MALE AND FEMALE SEXUAL PROBLEMS

Lack of sexual desire or arousal can affect both men and women and may stem from many different causes. Relationship problems (especially poor communication), stress, fear of failure, and maintaining old habits or patterns of sexual behaviour that are no longer satisfying can act as a barrier to intimacy and prevent men and women from responding sexually to each other. Managing stress levels, for example with massage techniques (see Chapter 5) and meditation and deep-breathing methods (see Chapter 10) may help. Both medicinal and recreational drugs can lead to sexual problems in men and women. Initially, alcohol in particular can seem to aid arousal by releasing inhibitions, but when used to excess, can inhibit sexual performance and may even cause long-term physical problems (see box, below).

Sensate focus

A therapist may recommend sensate focus. This teaches couples how to relax in each other's company, overcome performance anxiety and be intimate, without feeling pressurized to fulfil a goal. It is carried out in stages. In stage one, the couple take turns to touch each other in a sensitive and loving way, keeping to non-sexual areas of the body. It is important not to rush this stage. The couple do this twice a week, initially for 20 minutes and build up to 60 minutes over the next eight sessions.

At first, there is no talking. The couple concentrate on touching, stroking and caressing each other, enjoying the feel of their partner's body and, when it is their turn, gaining pleasure from their partner's touch. After two weeks, the breasts may be included and the couple will be encouraged to experiment with new sensations, for example, by using feathers, scented oils, simple sex toys or different fabrics.

After four weeks, the couple may move on to stage two. They will continue as before, but also explore and caress each other simultaneously, focusing on the sensations of being touched and touching. Later, they may include the genitals, stopping short of sexual arousal, and then progress to mutual masturbation and orgasm.

In stage three, the couple continue as in stage one and two, and then progress to penetration, but without movement. Over the next few sessions, they can include gentle thrusting movements and, finally, continue to orgasm – if that is what they both want. By this stage, the couple should be capable of loving, unhurried, unpressurized sex, with each partner keen to give pleasure as well as receive it, and not worried if lovemaking stops short of climax.

sex and drugs

Recreational drugs, such as alcohol, nicotine, cannabis and hard drugs, can cause sexual dysfunction in men and women, especially when used to excess. Medications linked with sexual disorders include anticonvulsants, antidepressants, antihypertensives, diuretics, and over-the-counter remedies for colds and insomnia. See your doctor if you think your medication may be the cause of a sexual problem. (Bear in mind that the disorder for which you're being treated may also cause sexual dysfunction.)

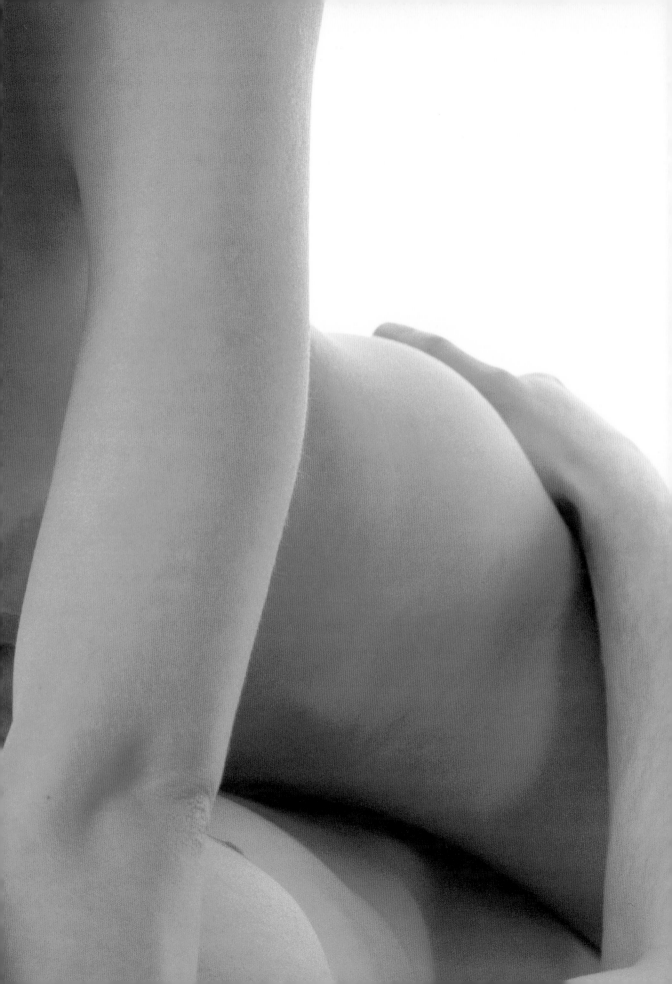

PLAYING SAFE

14

SEX IS THE MOST FUN TWO ADULTS CAN HAVE ON THEIR OWN. HOWEVER, THOSE

WHO WANT TO PLAY GROWN-UP GAMES MUST ABIDE BY GROWN-UP RULES.

UNPROTECTED SEX, ESPECIALLY WITH SOMEONE WHOSE SEXUAL HISTORY IS

UNKNOWN TO YOU, CAN LEAD TO AN UNPLANNED PREGNANCY AND RISKS YOUR

HEALTH, FERTILITY – AND POSSIBLY EVEN YOUR LIFE.

CHOOSING CONTRACEPTION

Today, there's a wide range of contraceptive methods to choose from, most for women's use. Your doctor can help you decide which method is best for you, taking into account your age and medical history. Hormonal and barrier methods are widely used, but there are other types. Most have a high success rate, if used correctly, and few side effects or risks. Emergency contraception is available for women up to five days after they've had unprotected sex – or think their method of contraception may have failed. Men and women can also choose sterilization as a form of contraception. However, this should be regarded as permanent and raises complex issues beyond the scope of this book.

HORMONAL METHODS

These mimic the natural release of the hormones oestrogen and/or progesterone produced at high levels in a pregnant woman. By taking hormones, a woman's body is tricked into acting as if it is pregnant and alters in such a way that pregnancy is not possible. Two widely-used hormonal methods are the oral combined pill, which contains oestrogen and a progestogen (synthetic progesterone), and the progestogen-only pill (POP) or mini-pill. Combined pills must be taken according to a strict 21- or 28-day regime (with either seven pill-free days or seven dummy pills). The POP must be taken every day within the same three-hour period. If the correct regime is not followed, protection may fail. Long-term hormonal contraception, containing a progestogen, is available. Injectable types protect against pregnancy for eight to 12 weeks, and implants (small capsules or rods inserted under the skin of the upper arm) provide up to five years' protection.

- **Advantages: Convenient and reliable. Allows spontaneity in lovemaking. Some types alleviate or protect against gynaecological disorders, including pelvic inflammatory disease (PID) [US: upper genital tract infection].**

- **Disadvantages: No protection against sexually transmitted diseases (STDs). Some types can have side effects and carry health risks, and may not be suitable for older women, diabetics, the overweight, smokers, and those with a history of heart disease, high blood pressure or blood clots. Your doctor will advise. Regular medical checks are required.**

BARRIER METHODS

These prevent sperm from reaching and fertilizing the egg. The most widely-used barrier method is the male condom, a latex or plastic

tip

Condoms not only protect against sexually transmitted diseases (STDs), including HIV, herpes, gonorrhoea, syphilis and chlamydia, they also reduce the risk of cervical cancer.

avoid petroleum products

Use only water-based lubricants if using latex condoms. Avoid lubricants and other products (such as baby oils and antifungal creams) containing petroleum as these damage latex condoms and make them ineffective. Plastic (polyurethane) condoms are not affected by petroleum.

contraception and reliability

Most contraceptive methods have a high reliability rating, based on how many women out of 100 might become pregnant if they use that method for a year. As a guide, unprotected sex has a rating of only 20 per cent. (In other words, 80 out of 100 women would get pregnant after a year of regular sex without using any contraception.)

METHOD	RELIABILITY (%)
Combined pill, hormone injection/implants	98–9
IUD/Progestogen-only pill	97–8
Male/female condom (plus spermicide)	97–8
Cap/diaphragm (plus spermicide)	97–8
Sponge (plus spermicide)	94–6
Natural birth control (used on its own) *	85–90
Post-coital pill	80
Spermicide (used on its own)**	75
No contraception	20

* Natural birth control is more reliable if a fertility monitor is used and it is combined with a barrier method during the fertile time of the month.

** It is not recommended that spermicide be used on its own.

(polyurethane) sheath that fits over a man's erect penis. To be effective, the man must withdraw his penis from his partner's vagina soon after ejaculating, before he loses his erection, or the condom may slip off. The female condom is larger and fits inside the vagina, with an inner ring that rests against the cervix and an outer ring that lies flat against the labia. It can be left in place for a little longer than the male condom as it is not held in place by the man's erection. For added protection, condoms may be combined with spermicide (see below).

There are many other forms of barrier contraception now available. These include the sponge, which fits inside the vagina; the diaphragm, covering the whole of the cervix (neck of the uterus); and the cap, which covers the cervical opening and is held in place by suction. A doctor or nurse fits the diaphragm or cap and teaches the woman how to insert it herself. The sponge, diaphragm and cap must all be used with a spermicidal cream, foam or gel containing a sperm-killing agent (such as nonoxynol-9) and left in place for six hours after intercourse.

fact

In 1995 almost half (48 per cent) of pregnancies in the USA were unintended. Many that were 'intended' were not planned or prepared for.

pill problems

If you forget to take a contraceptive pill, take it as soon as you remember, then take the next one at your usual time and use barrier contraception for the next seven days. You may need to skip the dummy pills or pill-free days and start with the next active pill (if unsure, a doctor or pharmacist can advise you). This advice also applies if you suffer vomiting or severe diarrhoea while taking the pill. Certain medications, including some antibiotics, barbiturates and anticonvulsants, can render the pill ineffective. Always tell a doctor or other healthcare professional if you're taking medication and/or using hormonal contraception.

- Stop taking the combined pill and consult a doctor immediately if you suffer severe breathlessness (or cough up blood), prolonged headaches, severe pain in the chest, stomach or leg, disturbed vision or hearing, or generalized itching.

Spermicides must be renewed before each sex act, or after three hours. Spermicidal pessaries [US: vaginal suppositories] can be used with the condom or diaphragm. They take ten to 30 minutes to dissolve.

- **Advantages: Reliable. Condoms protect against sexually transmitted diseases (STDs). Few side effects and few health risks.**

- **Disadvantages: Limited spontaneity in lovemaking. Condoms may cause reduced sensitivity. Caps and diaphragms carry a slight risk of toxic shock syndrome if left in for more than 24 hours. Some spermicides may cause a mild allergic reaction.**

IUD

The intra-uterine device (IUD or 'coil') is a small plastic device, usually wrapped in copper wire. Some types release progestogen. The IUD is inserted into the uterus by a doctor and left in place for one to eight years. It makes the uterus hostile to sperm, preventing ovulation and preventing a fertilized egg from attaching itself to the wall of the uterus. While the IUD carries a slight risk of pelvic inflammatory disease (PID) and infertility, the risk is lower for women in monogamous relationships.

- **Advantages: Convenient and reliable. Allows spontaneity in lovemaking. Some types provide limited protection against sexually transmitted diseases (STDs).**

- **Disadvantages: Can cause discomfort and bleeding. Slight risk of PID, infertility and ectopic pregnancy (embryo growing outside the uterus). Requires regular medical checks.**

NATURAL BIRTH CONTROL

This method requires that a woman learns how to recognize the days during her monthly menstrual cycle when she is fertile. She then abstains from having penetrative sex at this time, or uses a barrier method of contraception. Some women prefer this method for religious reasons or because they want to be more in tune with the natural rhythms of their bodies; others choose not to use hormones or mechanical methods. The signs indicating their fertile time include changes to the cervix, the appearance of increasing amounts of a slippery, stretchy and clear form of cervical mucus inside the vagina (at other times the mucus is absent or sticky, cloudy and thick), a slight rise in temperature (0.2–0.4°C) noticed first thing in the morning that lasts for three days (detected using a special thermometer), and

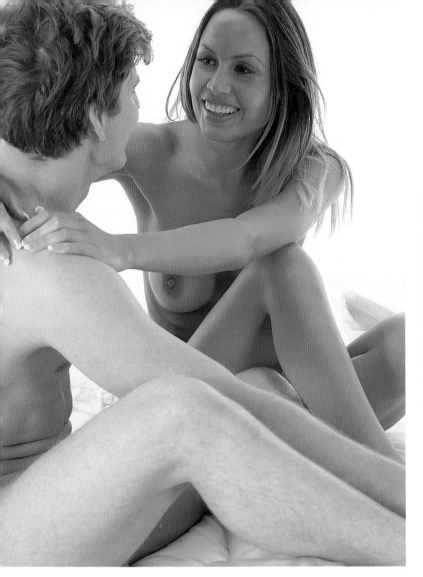

Any man or woman worth making love to will not need to be convinced or persuaded of the importance of safer sex.

further advice on diseases

Seek medical advice if you're unsure about your (or your partner's) sexual health, or there is any risk that you may have been infected. The following symptoms may indicate an STD, but some infections show no symptoms, especially in the early stages, yet still put your health and fertility at risk:

- **Abnormal discharge from the penis or vagina.**

- **Pain, soreness, redness or itching around the genital or anal area.**

- **Pain during sex or when urinating.**

- **Pain in the lower abdomen.**

- **Painful sores around the mouth, genitals or anus.**

Free testing, treatment and advice is available at GUM (genito-urinary medicine) clinics. They are listed in the telephone directory under GU, GUM or STD. Treatment is confidential and you can remain anonymous.

sometimes ovulation pain. Fertility monitors are available that can detect the rise in pre-ovulation hormone levels (in a urine sample) and help improve the accuracy of natural birth control.

- Advantages: **No health risks or side effects. Helps a woman to become more in tune with her body's natural cycles. Avoids the use of hormones.**

- Disadvantages: **Requires training. High failure risk unless practised diligently (or combined with barrier contraception).**

EMERGENCY CONTRACEPTION

There are two types of emergency contraception currently available. The first, the post-coital or 'morning-after' pill, is a fairly reliable method of hormonal contraception that can be taken at any time within three days of unprotected sex (ideally within 12 hours). It's given in two doses

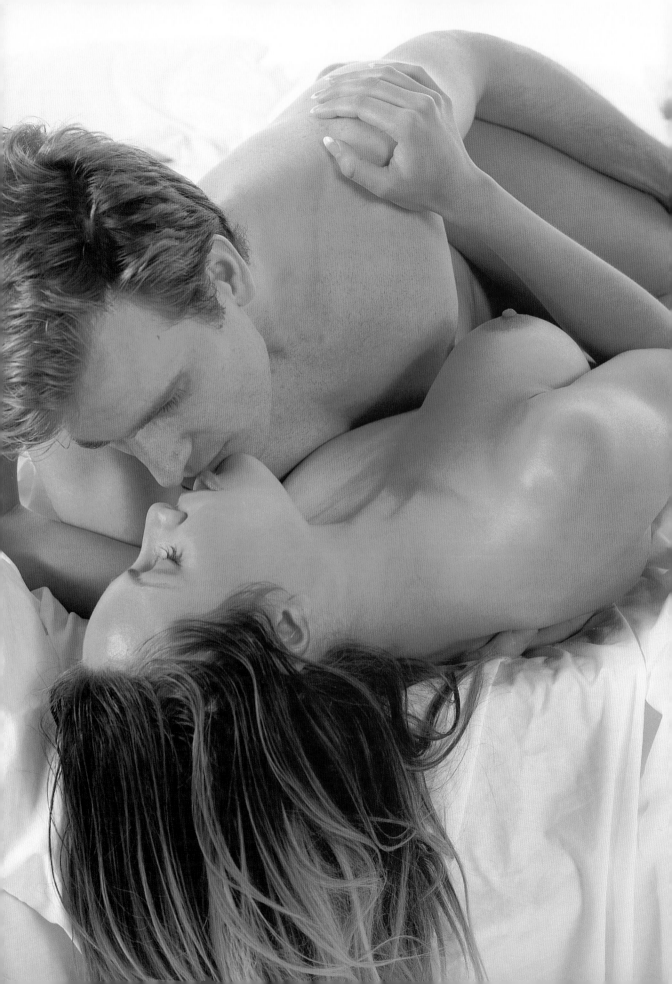

(one or two pills per dose), 12 hours apart, and it stops or delays the release of an egg, or prevents a fertilized egg attaching itself to the wall of the uterus. The second type, the IUD, is even more effective as emergency contraception and can be fitted within five days of unprotected sex (the sooner the better) or within five days of ovulation.

- **Advantages: Relatively safe back-up contraception if other methods are missed or fail. Many doctors now recommend keeping a pack of emergency contraception in reserve in case other methods fail.**

- **Disadvantages: The morning-after pill may cause minor side effects and is not as effective as long-term hormonal contraception. IUDs may not be suitable for all women.**

SAFER SEX

During the early stages of a sexual relationship you can't be sure of your partner's sexual history, so it's always wise to practise safer sex. This means modifying your behaviour to reduce the risk of contracting, or passing on, a sexually transmitted disease (STD). STDs can cause illness and infertility, and some are life-threatening.

Among the most common STDs are chlamydia (*Chlamydia trachomatis*), genital warts (*Human papillomavirus*), gonorrhoea (*Neisseria gonorrhoeae*), hepatitis A, B and C, herpes (*Herpes simplex I and II*), HIV (*Human immunodeficiency virus I and II* – the organisms that lead to acquired immune deficiency syndrome – or AIDS), syphilis (*Treponema pallidum*), Trichomoniasis (*Trichomonas vaginalis*), and Type II bacterial vaginosis (*Gardnerella vaginalis*).

Protection

It is not always possible to tell if a person is infected with an STD. In many cases, he or she may not display symptoms but may be capable of spreading the disease. You can reduce the risk of STDs by avoiding penetrative sex and practising, for example, mutual masturbation instead. Barrier methods of contraception – particularly male and female condoms – provide protection for penetrative sex, especially when used in conjunction with a spermicide (which kills many STD organisms).

Women, as well as men, should carry condoms in any situation that might lead to sex – even if lovemaking is not on the agenda. (The sexual urge is a powerful one that sweeps away the best intentions.) Use a condom for oral sex and to cover a vibrator, too.

PEACE OF MIND

Knowing you are fully protected will enable you to relax completely and really enjoy your lovemaking.

MEN AND CONDOMS

Some men are reluctant to use a condom, perhaps because of the slight loss of sensitivity it can cause, or simply because they prefer to leave contraception to their partners. But there are good reasons why a man who is not in a monogamous relationship should always wear a condom for penetrative sex. It helps to prevent the spread of sexually transmitted diseases; it shows he is willing to share responsibility for contraception, and it's a safeguard in case other methods fail. (In many countries, men have a financial, as well as a moral, responsibility for the children they father.) If her partner is reluctant to use a condom, a woman can suggest putting it on for him – and make it part of the foreplay. He'll enjoy the feeling of her hands on his penis and she can have fun touching and teasing him as she does it (see box, opposite).

ANAL SEX

While often regarded as a practice limited to male homosexuals, some heterosexual couples also practise anal sex. It carries an increased risk of spreading STDs because of the much greater chance of damage to the delicate tissues of the anus, giving viruses an easy route into the body. If the woman is willing to participate, she should ensure that her partner always wears a condom even if they are in a monogamous relationship. Thicker condoms, specially designed for anal sex, are available. The man should respect his partner's wishes and not coerce her into any practice she feels uncomfortable with and should be prepared to withdraw if she requests him to do so.

safety first

Even if the new man in your life seems perfect, for safety's sake, take precautions, especially if you decide to have sex on a first date.

• Do have the number of a reputable taxi firm with you – plus the fare – if you are away from home.

• Do limit your drinking. Excess alcohol leads to risky behaviour that you may later regret.

• Do carry condoms and insist on using them if you choose to have sex.

• Don't leave your drink unattended. It is easy to spike an alcoholic drink by lacing it with a hypnotic drug or strong liquor.

• Don't agree to practices such as bondage that leave you vulnerable.

• Don't be rushed into anything you're not ready for. Any man worth making love to will be sensitive to your feelings.

• Don't hesitate to leave if you feel uneasy about a situation.

putting on a condom

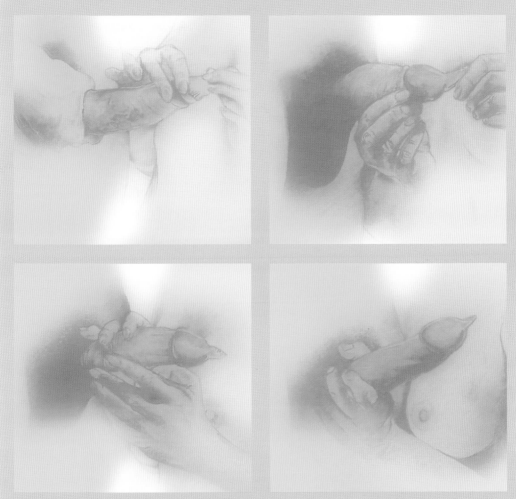

When removing a condom from its package, take care not to tear it with your nails or jewellery. If it gets damaged, throw it away and use another one. Always use a new condom for each act of intercourse and check the expiry date on the package first.

- Squeeze the air out of the teat at the end and place the condom on the tip of the erect penis. Still holding the teat, start to unroll the condom over the penis, taking care not to stretch it too tightly or damage it with your nails.

- Roll the condom down to the base. If the erection begins to weaken, give the penis a swift rub. After ejaculation, hold the base of the condom as the penis is withdrawn to prevent semen from spilling out.

FURTHER READING

Adler, MW, *ABC of Sexually Transmitted Diseases*, London, BMJ Books, 1998.

Clubb, E and Knight J, *Fertility – A Comprehensive Guide to Natural Family Planning*, Devon, David & Charles, 1992.

Cooper, C, Cooper, R and Eakin L, *Living with Stress*, London, Penguin Books, 1988.

Desmond, K (ed), *Reader's Digest Guide to Love & Sex*, London, Reader's Digest Association, 1998.

Hawton, K, 'Treatment of sexual dysfunctions by sex therapy and other approaches', Br J Psychiatry, 1995; 167:307–14.

Lacroix, N, *Love, Sex & Intimacy*, London, Anness Publishing, 1995.

Litvinoff, S, *Relate Guide to Loving Relationships*, London, Ebury Press, 1992.

Masters, WH, Johnson VE and Kolodny, RC, *Human Sexuality*, New York, HarperCollins, 1995.

Mehta, DK (ed), *British National Formulary*, London, BMA/RPS of GB, 2001.

Meston, C, 'Instruments designed to assess female sexual function'. In: 'Female Sexual Function Forum: New Perspectives in The Management of Female Sexual Dysfunction', Boston University School of Medicine, Department of Urology; October 2000; page 184.

Sayle, AE et al., 'Sex in late pregnancy does not generally increase risk of preterm delivery', Obstet & Gynecol 2001; 97: 283–9.

Tomlinson, JM (ed), *ABC of Sexual Health*, London, BMJ Books, 1999.

USEFUL CONTACTS

UK
Sexual Health
Blackliners
Unit 4–6 Eurolink Business Centre
49 Effra Road
London SW2 1BZ
helpline: 020 7738 5274
www.blackliners.org
(Support and information on sexual health for black people)

British Pregnancy Advisory Service (BPAS)
Austy Manor
Wootton Wawen
Solihull
West Midlands B95 6X
tel: 01564 793225
fax: 01564 794935
BPAS Actionline (for appointments):
0845 7304030
(open seven days a week)
www.bpas.org
(BPAS was established as a registered charity in 1968 to provide a safe, legal abortion service. It is now Britain's largest single abortion provider. To book an appointment at any of the consultation centres throughout the UK, call the national Actionline (above). Other services include pregnancy testing, crisis pregnancy counselling, emergency contraception and after-abortion support)

Brook Advisory Centres
tel: 020 7617 8000
(24-hour helpline with recorded information for young people)

Contraceptive Education Service
helpline: 020 7837 4044
(England and Wales);
0141 576 5088 (Scotland);
028 9032 5488 (Northern Ireland)

London Lesbian & Gay Switchboard
tel: 020 7837 7324
(24-hour helpline)

National AIDS Helpline
tel: 0800 567123 (24-hour helpline);
0800 521 361 (24-hour minicom for the hard-of-hearing)
(General advice and information on sexually transmitted diseases)

Terrence Higgins Trust
52–4 Grays Inn Road
London WC1X 8JU
helpline: 020 7242 1010
(from 12 noon to 10 pm every day)
www.tht.org.uk
(Counselling and advice on sexually transmitted diseases)

General Health
Institute for Complementary Medicine (ICM)
21 Portland Place
London W1N 3AF
tel: 020 7237 5165
www.icmedicine.co.uk
(Write, enclosing a large SAE, for information on courses and practitioners)

Men's Health Helpline
tel: 020 8995 4448
(Medical advisory service every Monday, Tuesday and Thursday from 7–9 pm)

Women's Health Concern
helpline: 01628 483612
(Help and advice on female health problems)

Sexual/Relationship Problems
British Association for Counselling & Psychotherapy (BACP)
1 Regent Place
Rugby CV21 2PJ
tel: 0870 4435252
www.counselling.co.uk
(Write, enclosing a large SAE, for a list of local therapists or centres)

The Impotence Association
PO Box 10296
London SW17 9WH
helpline: 020 8767 7791
(Open 9–5 pm, Monday–Friday)
www.impotence.org.uk
(Counselling and advice on male and female sexual dysfunction)

The Institute of Psychosexual Medicine
12 Chandos Street
Cavendish Square
London W1G 9BZ
tel: 020 7580 0631
(Write, enclosing a large SAE, for a list of accredited doctors)

Relate
Herbert Gray College
Little Church Street
Rugby
CV21 3AP
tel: 01788 573241
fax: 01788 535007
www.relate.org.uk
(Relationship counselling and
psychosexual therapy)

Stockists

Ann Summers
Head Office
Gadoline House
2 Godstone Road
Whyteleafe
Surrey CR3 0EA
tel: 020 8645 8320
(for stockists or to book a party)
www.annsummers.com
(The UK's unique passion and fashion
retailer – providing everything from
luscious fashion-led lingerie to love
oils and body paints, from PVC and
playwear to sex toys and novelties)

Janet Reger International Limited
2 Beauchamp Place
London SW3 1NJ
tel: 020 7584 9360
www.janetreger.com
(Luxurious lingerie)

Neals Yard Remedies
26–34 Ingate Place
Battersea
London SW8 3NS
tel: 020 7627 1949
(Customer Services in UK and Europe)
mail order: 0161 831 7875 (UK)
fax: 020 7498 2505
www.nealsyardremedies.com
(Aromatherapy products, herbal
remedies and homoeopathy)

USA

Gay Men's Health Crisis (GMHC)
hotline: 001 212 807 6655
(Counselling for heterosexual and
homosexual men on all aspects of
sexual health)

Heart to Heart Counseling Centers
PO Box 5
1055 Colorado Springs,
Co. 80949
http://www.sexaddict.com
(Support for sex addicts – newsletter,

support group links, religious links
and practical advice for the partners
of sex addicts)

The Kinsey Institute for Research in Sex,
Gender and Reproduction
Indiana University
Bloomington
IN 47405
tel: 001 812 855 7686
www.indiana.edu/~kinsey
(Promotes interdisciplinary research
and scholarship in the field of human
sexuality. Access to The Kinsey
Institute's own sexual clinic, information
services, research, publications, library
and other sexology links)

Neals Yard Remedies
tel: 001 213 746 5363
(US distributor)
www.nealsyardremedies.com
(Aromatherapy products, herbal
remedies and homoeopathy)

San Francisco AIDS Foundation
tel: 001 415 863 2437

Sex on the Web

The Alan Guttmacher Institute
www.agi-USA.org
(Research and information on family
planning, sexual health, sexually
transmitted diseases, abortion and
related topics)

All About Sex
http://www.allaboutsex.org
A discussion website for teens and
their parents on the first time, getting
caught, protection, censorship, sexual
development, virginity, experimentation
and homosexuality.

Cosmopolitan: Cosmos Sex Lessons
http://cosmo.women.com/cos/love/index.htm
(*Cosmopolitan* magazine's online sex
expert answers your questions; features
on love and sex, and what's hot)

Enjoying Safer Sex
http://aids.about.com/health/aids/cs/safesex
(Advice on responsible sex; also
gay/lesbian issues, men's and
women's health matters)

The G-Zone
http://doctorg.com/FemaleEjaculation.htm
(Female sexuality)

Men's Health Guide to Sex
and Relationships
www.menshealth.com/sex_relationships
(Help, tips and suggestions on sex,
women, positions and sex games)

Nerve Magazine
http://www.nerve.com
Online erotic print magazine with
thoughtful articles, short stories and
photos for men and woman.
Includes position of the day and
celebrity 'first-time' essays.

Seniors-Site.com
http://seniors-site.com/sex/
Sexual information, articles and
products for seniors on better sex,
protection and sexual dysfunction.

Sex-tips Directory for Adult Men
and Women
http://www.sex-tips.com/sextips/
Manuals (safer sex, meeting singles),
shopping (sex apparel) and advice.

Sex Therapy Online
www.sexology.org
(Access to the finest sexologists and
sex therapists in the world)

Sexual Harassment and
Rape Resources
http://www.igc.apc.org/women/activist/harass.html

Sexual Harassment State Hotlines
http://www.feminist.org/911/harass.html

Thirdage
http://www.thirdage.com/romance/
Love and sex advice, quizzes and
ideas for romance and seduction for
adults in their forties and fifties.

PICTURE CREDITS

All photographs by Peter Pugh-Cook
except for the following:
Carlton Books Ltd./Ken Niven: 12,
21, 53tr; C Harvey & T Belshaw:
10, 66, 68tl, 68bl, 107r; Alan
Randall: 40, 41, 42, 43, 44, 48,
53, 84, 106/7; Susannah Price:
45; Alistair Hughes: 15, 51, 52,
66, 85t, 86b, 87t, 91, 93t, 105.

INDEX

Figures in italics indicate captions.

ACKNOWLEDGEMENTS

The author would like to pay a special tribute to William H Masters, who died in the year this book was produced. As one of the great pioneers of sex research, with his wife, Virginia E Johnson, he did so much to shed light on a badly-neglected area of human experience. Special thanks are due to Peter Pugh-Cook, the photographer, and models Ricky Dearman and Janie Dickens for their enthusiasm, Katrina Dallamore and Bobby Birchall at DW Design for inspired art direction, Anwar Jones, fitness instructor at Rowans, Finsbury Park, London, for checking the 'sexercises', and to my editor, Jane Donovan, for her much-appreciated support and encouragement.